CW01660976

SBAs for the Part 1 MRCOG

Andrew Sizer and Neil Chapman

SBAs for the Part 1 MRCOG

A Guide to Single Best Answer Questions for the Part 1 MRCOG Examination

RCOG PRESS

© 2012 ROYAL COLLEGE OF OBSTETRICIANS AND GYNAECOLOGISTS

First published 2012

All rights reserved. No part of this publication may be reproduced, stored or transmitted in any form or by any means, without the prior written permission of the publisher or, in the case of reprographic reproduction, in accordance with the terms of licences issued by the Copyright Licensing Agency in the UK [www.cla.co.uk]. Enquiries concerning reproduction outside the terms stated here should be sent to the publisher at the UK address printed on this page.

Registered names: The use of registered names, trademarks, etc. in this publication does not imply, even in the absence of a specific statement, that such names are exempt from the relevant laws and regulations and therefore free for general use.

Product liability: Drugs and their doses are mentioned in this text. While every effort has been made to ensure the accuracy of the information contained within this publication, neither the authors nor the publishers can accept liability for errors or omissions. The final responsibility for delivery of the correct dose remains with the physician prescribing and administering the drug. In every individual case the respective user must check current indications and accuracy by consulting other pharmaceutical literature and following the guidelines laid down by the manufacturers of specific products and the relevant authorities in the country in which they are practising.

The rights of Andrew Sizer and Neil Chapman to be identified as Authors of this work have been asserted by them in accordance with the Copyright, Designs and Patents Act, 1988.

A machine-readable catalogue record for this publication is available from the British Library [www.bl.uk/catalogue/listings.html]

ISBN 978-1-906985-58-5

DAMAGED

Published by the **RCOG Press** at the
Royal College of Obstetricians and Gynaecologists
27 Sussex Place, Regent's Park
London NW1 4RG

Registered Charity No. 213280

RCOG Press is a trademark of the Royal College of Obstetricians and Gynaecologists

Cover image © Gary Buss/Taxi/Getty Images

Illustrations by Oxford Designers & Illustrators; © RCOG

Image on page 99 reproduced from: Kanaya H et al. Successful monozygotic twin delivery following in vitro maturation of oocytes retrieved from a woman with polycystic ovary syndrome: case report. *Hum Reprod* 2006;21(7):1777–80, by permission of Oxford University Press.

RCOG Press Editor: Claire Dunn

Design and typesetting: FiSH Books, Enfield

Printed by Latimer Trend and Co. Ltd., Estover Road, Plymouth PL6 7PL

Contents

Preface

The successful completion of examinations leading to Membership of the Royal College of Obstetricians and Gynaecologists is a mandatory requirement to complete specialist training in the UK.

The Membership examination consists of two parts: Part 1, traditionally thought of as a basic science examination, and Part 2, a clinical examination. However, both parts of the examination have undergone significant change over the past few years to take into account developments in practice and knowledge as well as new ideas in medical education and assessment.

From the March 2012 sitting of the examination, there will be some significant changes to the Part 1 examination. Changes to the curriculum and syllabus have been approved by the General Medical Council, resulting in an examination that will test applied basic and clinical sciences in addition to the traditional theoretical component. Another significant change to the examination is the introduction of 'single best answer questions', which replace the extended matching questions that have previously been used.

This book clarifies the new structure of the examination and provides many examples of the new single best answer question format.

About the authors

Andrew Sizer is a Consultant in Obstetrics and Gynaecology at the Shrewsbury and Telford Hospitals NHS Trust. He has a special interest in reproductive medicine and surgery. He is also Senior Lecturer and Undergraduate Lead for Women's Health at the Shropshire Campus of Keele University School of Medicine. Mr Sizer is co-convenor of the RCOG Part 1 MRCOG Revision course and served on the Part 1 MRCOG Sub-committee from 2008 to 2011. He was appointed as a Part 2 MRCOG examiner in 2011. He graduated from the University of Wales College of Medicine in 1994, having completed an intercalated BSc and PhD in Physiology. He then undertook an MD in male infertility and completed his specialist training in 2005. He worked for a year at Kilimanjaro Christian Medical College in Tanzania, from 2001 to 2002.

Neil Chapman is a non-clinical Lecturer in Reproductive Medicine in the Academic Unit of Reproductive and Developmental Medicine at the University of Sheffield. His laboratory research focuses on understanding how the myometrial genome is regulated by NF-κB during pregnancy and labour. The principal funding for this work is currently provided by the Medical Research Council and the Wellcome Trust. He was a member of the Part 1 MRCOG Sub-committee from 2007 to 2011 and was engaged in developing both extended matching questions and, more recently, single best answer questions, which form the basis of the new Part 1 examination. Dr Chapman graduated from the University of Sheffield with a BSc (Hons) in Biochemistry and Physiology in 1994 and a PhD in Molecular and Reproductive Biology in 1997. He has been a Fellow of the Higher Education Academy since 2008.

Acknowledgements

The authors would like to acknowledge the assistance of the following colleagues in the development of this book:

Mr Paul Carter, St George's Hospital, London

Mr Nigel Davies, University Hospital of Wales

Dr Claudine Domoney, Chelsea and Westminster Hospital

Dr Raji Ganesan, Birmingham Women's Hospital

Mr Anthony Griffiths, University Hospital of Wales

Mr Adam Gornall, Royal Shrewsbury Hospital

Dr Alex Landau, RCOG

Dr Michele Mohajer, Royal Shrewsbury Hospital

Professor Neil Pugh, Cardiff University

Professor Peter Soothill, University of Bristol

Abbreviations

α-FP	alpha fetoprotein
AIS	androgen insensitivity syndrome
APC	activated protein C
ATP	adenosine triphosphate
BMI	body mass index
BRCA1	breast cancer gene 1
CA125	cancer antigen 125
Ca^{2+}	calcium ions
cAMP	cyclic adenosine monophosphate
cGMP	cyclic guanosine monophosphate
CTG	cardiotocograph
DEXA	dual-energy X-ray absorptiometry
DHEA	dehydroepiandrosterone
DVT	deep vein thrombosis
EMQ	extended matching question
FSH	follicle-stimulating hormone
gamma GT	gamma-glutamyl transferase
GBS	group B Streptococcus
GnRH	gonadotrophin-releasing hormone
GP	general practitioner
hCG	human chorionic gonadotrophin
HLA	human leucocyte antigen
H-P-O	hypothalamic–pituitary–ovarian
HPV	human papillomavirus
HSG	hysterosalpingography
IFN-γ	interferon gamma

Ig	immunoglobulin
IP3	inositol-1,4,5,-triphosphate
IV	intravenous
IVF	in vitro fertilisation
LH	luteinising hormone
MCQ	multiple choice question
MHC	major histocompatibility complex
MRI	magnetic resonance imaging
NK	natural killer
NO	nitric oxide
NSAID	non-steroidal anti-inflammatory drug
PCO_2	partial pressure of carbon dioxide
PCOS	polycystic ovary syndrome
PO_2	partial pressure of oxygen
RCOG	Royal College of Obstetricians and Gynaecologists
RhD	rhesus D
SBA	single best answer question
SHBG	sex hormone-binding globulin
SIADH	syndrome of inappropriate antidiuretic hormone
STD	sexually transmitted disease
STI	sexually transmitted infection
T_4	thyroxine
TGFβ	transforming growth factor beta
TSH	thyroid-stimulating hormone
VEGF	vascular endothelial growth factor
WHO	World Health Organization

Foreword

The Part 1 MRCOG examination is a summative, primary assessment of the knowledge and understanding of the basic science principles which are relevant to the practice of obstetrics and gynaecology. This knowledge of the principles of basic science is important; these principles constitute the 'building blocks' of further knowledge and clinical judgement. However, we are increasingly aware of the role the Part 1 examination fulfils as an assessment of clinical competence in the early years of training. The aim of achieving a more effective balance between coverage of basic science content and relevance to clinical duties has resulted in a change to the Part 1 MRCOG from March 2012. The change will entail a shift of emphasis to make the examination more relevant to the continuing learning and development objectives of the specialty training programme.

This book is to aid those sitting the new-style Part 1 examination. The introduction to the single best answer format, with examples of how this question format interacts with the syllabus, should help all those attempting the Part 1 MRCOG examination.

Nigel Davies
Chair, Examination and Assessment Committee, RCOG

How to use this book

Chapter 1 of this book provides an overview of the new syllabus and curriculum for the Part 1 MRCOG examination, and also explains the structure of single best answer questions (SBAs) and the rationale for using this question format in the Part 1 MRCOG examination.

Chapter 2 outlines the syllabus topics in the Part 1 MRCOG blue-printing matrix for paper 1 of the examination and provides example questions from all relevant areas; that is, from the logbook core modules and the subject domains. Chapter 3 is identical in format to chapter 2, but covers the syllabus areas relevant to paper 2 of the examination.

Chapter 4 provides a mock paper for paper 1 of the examination, and chapter 5 provides a mock paper for paper 2 of the examination.

Appendix 1 contains the blueprinting matrix for the examination. Appendix 2 contains an example answer sheet for the SBA component of the examination. Appendix 3 provides answers to the sample questions in chapter 2, appendix 4 provides answers to the questions in chapter 3, appendix 5 provides answers to the questions in chapter 4 and appendix 6 provides answers to the questions in chapter 5.

1 | Structure and content of the Part 1 MRCOG examination

From March 2012, there will be some significant changes to both the syllabus and examination style for the Part 1 MRCOG examination. These changes have been ratified by the General Medical Council and aim to produce an examination that is more relevant to the 21st century trainee aspiring to have a career in obstetrics and gynaecology.

Essentially, the changes to the Part 1 MRCOG entail a shift of emphasis to ensure that the examination continues to provide a relevant foundation for the continuation of learning and the development objectives of the specialty training programme. This change has required a realignment of the proportional contribution of existing areas of the Part 1 MRCOG syllabus and a revised blueprinting exercise that references explicitly the modules of the core curriculum against the existing global question domains. The modification of the existing examination format will ensure that this revised syllabus coverage can be tested appropriately to reflect the new desired emphasis of the Part 1 MRCOG.

The new Part 1 MRCOG contains questions that are clearly relevant to an applied sciences examination in obstetrics and gynaecology, with less of a focus on de-contextualised fundamental science. In essence, the new examination still requires candidates to have a robust understanding of fundamental science, both physical and biomedical, which will serve as a foundation on which to build subsequent clinical knowledge. The major difference from the previous examination is that knowledge is tested in a more clinical context to ensure candidates have the appropriate knowledge to function as specialty trainees on a daily basis. This knowledge is tested using a mixture of single best answer questions (SBAs) and true/false multiple choice questions (MCQs).

Rationale for single best answer questions

Until March 2007, the Part 1 MRCOG examination consisted of two papers each containing 300 true/false MCQs. Extended matching questions (EMQs) were then introduced, with each paper containing 20 EMQs and 240 MCQs. EMQs have been demonstrated to test understanding and application of knowledge better than MCQs and are certainly more reliable individually in differentiating between good and poor candidates. Although MCQ papers produce reliable assessments by testing a wide range of knowledge in a relatively short time period, there is some concern that they merely test recall of facts without context rather than the candidate's understanding of a given subject. The obvious corollary, therefore, is that one could ask: if EMQs are a good assessment tool, then why change?

The advantage of SBAs over EMQs is that they assess understanding and knowhow rather than mere factual knowledge, but in a shorter period of time. As such, more SBAs can be included within an examination, allowing a wider number of subject areas to be tested without compromising the applied nature of the knowledge being assessed. This also allows the number of MCQs to be reduced so that the focus of the examination is understanding rather than factual recall. It will also reduce the 'guess' element to the examination: the chances of a 'wild guess' being correct in an MCQ question is 50%, whereas in an SBA it is only 20%. As such, SBAs combine the benefits of both EMQs (testing of more complex knowledge) and MCQs (increased assessment scope within a given time period). Indeed, the SBA format is being used increasingly by other medical royal colleges as well as by the General Medical Council.

SBAs for the Part 1 MRCOG are written by members of the Part 1 MRCOG Sub-Committee. New questions are scrutinised carefully by the whole committee to ensure they pass a number of criteria: they are clinically relevant; the written English is of the highest standard, thereby avoiding ambiguity; and one answer is definitely the correct answer.

Structure of single best answer questions

Each SBA consists of three components:

- a stem (a clinical or scientific scenario)
- a 'lead-in' or question asking which is the single best answer
- five options, of which one is clearly the correct answer.

All questions are checked to ensure they pass the 'cover test'. This means that a good candidate should be able to cover the option list and, just by reading the stem, know what the correct answer is.

The Part 1 MRCOG syllabus

The syllabus has been mapped to the 19 modules of the core curriculum; note that modules 2, 4 and 19 are **not** examined in the Part 1 examination. A blueprinting matrix has also been developed that shows how the modules and the subject domains are related (Appendix 1).

There are now 14 subject domains that are tested in the examination, which is a change from the previous diet. There are two important new additions: 'data interpretation' and 'clinical management'. These sections cover aspects of interpretation of standard clinical data and laboratory analyses, and assess the candidate's understanding of the clinical management of common obstetric and gynaecological problems encountered at this level of training.

The most up-to-date details of the syllabus can be found on the RCOG website, which candidates are strongly advised to consult.

Structure of the Part 1 MRCOG examination

The examination is divided into two papers. Each paper contains 60 SBAs and 30 five-part true/false MCQs. The weighting for the SBA and true/false MCQ component of each paper is the same: 150 marks are available for each section. The time allowed to fully complete each paper is 2 hours 30 minutes (5 hours total examining time). Contrast this to the previous Part 1 MRCOG examination:

Previous format	Papers 1 and 2: 2 hours per paper	20 EMQs (60 marks) 48 five-part MCQs (240 marks)
Format from March 2012	Papers 1 and 2: 2 hours 30 minutes per paper	60 SBAs (150 marks) 30 five-part MCQs (150 marks)

Make sure that you leave enough time to fully complete the answer sheets, as this has to be done within the time frame of the examination. No time will be allowed to transfer answers if these have been written in draft form on the question paper.

Figure 1 demonstrates the approximate distribution of marks for each of the subject domains in the two papers, although candidates are advised that the breakdown will vary from sitting to sitting.

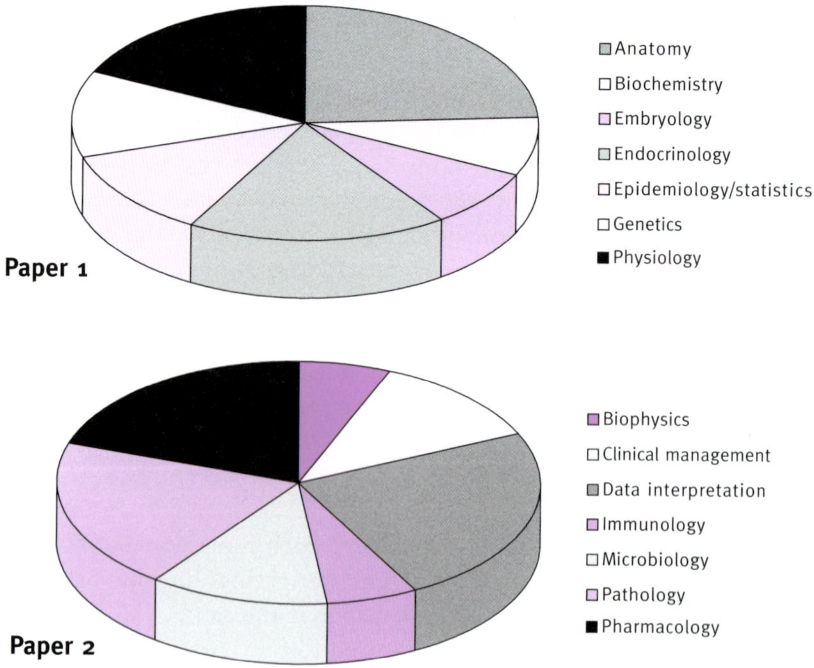

Figure 1 Distribution of marks by subject domain in papers 1 and 2

The blueprinting matrix that has been developed by the College is shown in Appendix 1. This shows in some detail how the modules and domains are inter-related and the subject areas that need to be covered in order to be properly prepared for the examination.

Examples of how different SBAs fit into the various areas of the blueprinting matrix are given in chapter 3.

Approach to answering single best answer questions

In many ways, the cover test is a good approach to answering SBAs, as the option lists may include many distractors which aim to deflect the uncertain candidate. It is often best, therefore, to cover over the options, read the stem and deduce what you think the correct answer is before looking at the option list. Obviously, if the answer you come up with is not on the list, there is clearly something wrong with your knowledge! However, if the answer you come up with is on the list, that is most likely to be the correct response. It is better to go with your first hunch and not be distracted by possible incorrect answers in the option list.

2 | Part 1 MRCOG blueprinting matrix, syllabus topics and example questions for paper 1

This chapter and chapter 3 break down the blueprinting matrix into individual components and provide example questions where appropriate.

Not all module and domain intersections on the matrix have a relevant syllabus subject area; for example, there are no syllabus topics for the Part 1 examination combining core module 3 (IT, governance and research) and the embryology domain. On the other hand, other syllabus areas may appear on the grid more than once.

The list of syllabus topics given here is not exhaustive. Obstetrics and gynaecology is a continually evolving subject and new knowledge is appearing all the time. Likewise, the Part 1 examination is also continually evolving. It is therefore wise to always consult the RCOG website (www.rcog.org.uk) for the most up-to-date syllabus and examination information.

Answers to the questions in this chapter can be found in appendix 3.

Anatomy domain

Core modules 5–7

Syllabus topics: Surgical anatomy of the pelvis and abdomen. Detailed functional anatomy of abdominal wall, abdominal cavity and pelvis, their contents, relevant bones, joints, muscles, blood vessels, lymphatics, nerve supply and histology. Understanding of breast and endocrine gland anatomy. Organisation and structure of the cell and its organelles. Classification systems for gynaecological and obstetric conditions.

SBA 1

During a caesarean section, the rectus sheath is divided to reveal the rectus muscle. The combined aponeuroses of which muscles form the anterior component of the rectus sheath?

A External and internal oblique
B External oblique and transversus abdominis
C Internal oblique and transversus abdominis
D Pyramidalis and serratus anterior
E Pyramidalis and transversus abdominis

Core module 8

Syllabus topics: Anatomical adaptations to pregnancy. Breast changes in pregnancy. Anatomical interpretation of fetal and maternal images from X-ray, ultrasound and magnetic resonance imaging.

SBA 2

The lactating breast is divided into lobules, each of which contains a lactiferous duct. Approximately how many lobules does each breast contain?

A 1
B 2
C 5
D 10
E 20

Core module 10

Syllabus topics: Obstetric anatomy of the pelvis and abdomen. Changes during late pregnancy and in labour. Mechanism of childbirth.

SBA 3

What type of joint is formed at the symphysis pubis?

A Cartilaginous
B Condyloid

C Fibrous
D Synarthrodial
E Synovial

Core module 12

Syllabus topic: Structural changes in the newborn.

SBA 4
Closure of the ductus arteriosus following lung inflation shortly after birth is mediated by which vasoactive substance?

A Bradykinin
B Prostacyclin
C Substance P
D Vasopressin
E VEGF

Core module 13

Syllabus topic: Gynaecological anatomy.

SBA 5
The uterine artery is a direct branch of which major artery in the pelvis?

A External iliac
B Internal iliac
C Femoral
D Obturator
E Pudendal

Core modules 14–16

Syllabus topics: Anatomy of the hypothalamus and pituitary, and the male and female reproductive organs. Surgical anatomy of the pelvis and abdomen.

SBA 6

The pituitary gland sits in a small bony cavity in the skull known as...?

A Diaphragma sellae
B Optic chiasm
C Sella turcica
D Sphenoid sinus
E Third ventricle

Core module 17

Syllabus topic: Anatomical changes relevant to tumours in the female.

SBA 7

A woman with advanced cervical cancer presents to hospital with worsening left loin pain. Which structure is most likely to have become obstructed?

A Cervix
B Ureter
C Urethra
D Uterine artery
E Vagina

Core module 18

Syllabus topic: Functional anatomy of the pelvic floor, kidney and urinary tract.

SBA 8

The motor supply of the levator ani muscle is derived predominantly from which spinal segment?

A L5
B S1
C S2
D S3
E S4

Endocrinology domain

Core modules 5–7

Syllabus topics: Mechanisms of hormone action. Hormone types. Peri-operative care and common endocrinopathies (e.g. diabetes and thyroid disorders). Effects of anaesthesia and surgery on endocrine homeostasis and fluid balance.

SBA 9

Which signalling mechanism involves the release of hormone from cells to act locally on other cells?

A Autocrine
B Endocrine
C Exocrine
D Metacrine
E Paracrine

Core module 8

Syllabus topics: Endocrinology of pregnancy. The placenta as an endocrine gland.

SBA 10

What is the major estrogen produced by the placenta during pregnancy?

A Dehydroepiandrosterone
B Estradiol
C Estriol
D Estrone
E Ethinylestradiol

Core module 9

Syllabus topics: Diabetes in pregnancy. Pituitary, thyroid, adrenal and other endocrine disorders relevant to pregnancy.

SBA 11

What percentage of pregnancies are complicated by gestational diabetes mellitus?

A <1%
B 1–5%
C 10–15%
D 20%
E 25%

Core module 10

Syllabus topics: Endocrinology of parturition. Development and maturation of the fetal endocrine system.

SBA 12

What is the earliest gestational age at which the fetal endocrine system is thought to be fully functional?

A 6/40
B 10/40
C 16/40
D 24/40
E 30/40

Core module 12

Syllabus topic: Endocrinology of lactation.

SBA 13

Hyperplasia and hypertrophy of alveolar cells in the breast during pregnancy are stimulated by which hormones?

A Estrone and hCG
B Human placental lactogen and estradiol
C Human placental lactogen and progesterone
D Prolactin and human placental lactogen
E Prolactin and progesterone

Core module 13

Syllabus topics: Menopause and endocrine effects on bone, vasomotor system, etc. Puberty and growth. Menstrual cycle.

SBA 14
A premature menopause is said to occur when the ovaries cease functioning before what age?

A 20 years
B 30 years
C 40 years
D 50 years
E 60 years

Core module 14

Syllabus topics: Endocrinology of the H-P-O axis. Endocrinopathies leading to anovulation in PCOS, hypogonadal hypogonadism, hyperprolactinaemia and premature ovarian failure.

SBA 15
A woman with schizophrenia presents to the clinic with galactorrhoea. What is the most likely cause of her hyperprolactinaemia?

A Hypothyroidism
B Macroprolactinoma
C Microprolactinoma
D Renal failure
E Use of phenothiazine drugs

Core module 15

Syllabus topic: Interactions between hormonal contraceptives and endocrine physiology.

SBA 16

A woman with polycystic ovaries and oligomenorrhoea commences the combined oral contraceptive pill to induce regular withdrawal bleeds. What will happen to her serum levels of FSH and SHBG?

	FSH	SHBG
A	Fall	Rise
B	Rise	Fall
C	Rise	Rise
D	Fall	Fall
E	No change	No change

Core module 16

Syllabus topic: Maternal recognition of pregnancy, endocrinology of the corpus luteum and early pregnancy.

SBA 17

What are the two major steroid hormones produced by the corpus luteum?

A Estradiol and hCG
B Estradiol and progesterone
C Estradiol and testosterone
D Progesterone and hCG
E Progesterone and testosterone

Core module 17

Syllabus topic: Hormone-secreting and hormone-dependent tumours in gynaecology.

SBA 18

Which substance has been used as a tumour marker for granulosa cell tumour of the ovary?

A Alphafetoprotein
B Estrone
C hCG
D Inhibin
E Progesterone

Physiology domain

Core module 1

Syllabus topic: Understand the physiological basis of physical signs in obstetrics and gynaecology.

SBA 19

A woman attending the antenatal clinic is concerned about a dark line that has appeared on her skin between the umbilicus and the pubic symphysis. You reassure her that this is a normal feature of pregnancy and is known as:

A Chloasma
B Linea alba
C Linea nigra
D Striae gravidarum
E Striae nigricans

Core modules 5–7

Syllabus topics: Physiology of wound healing. Physiology of major organ systems as applied to surgical practice. Fluid and electrolyte balance in the perioperative period. Nutritional physiology in health and disease. Principles of blood transfusion.

SBA 20

A woman who was known to be anaemic in pregnancy is noted to be pale and tachycardic after delivery. Her haemoglobin level is 6.2 g/dl. What is the most appropriate blood product for her?

A Fresh frozen plasma
B Frozen red cells
C Packed red cells
D Platelets
E Whole blood

Core module 8

Syllabus topics: Physiology of pregnancy including acid–base, fluid and electrolyte balance in healthy and pathological pregnancy. Fetal physiology and its development with fetal growth. Cellular physiology of the major organ systems in the non-pregnant woman.

SBA 21

By what percentage does cardiac output increase in pregnancy?

A 5%
B 10%
C 20%
D 40%
E 80%

Core module 9

Syllabus topic: Physiology in disorders of pregnancy.

SBA 22

A woman with a twin pregnancy attends an antenatal clinic at 35/40 gestation. She is experiencing intense itching but has no rash, pain or fever. What is the most likely diagnosis?

A Acute fatty liver of pregnancy

B Gallstones
C Hepatitis A
D Hepatitis B
E Obstetric cholestasis

Core module 10

Syllabus topics: Physiology of parturition, myometrial contractility and cervical dilatation. Fetal physiology in late pregnancy and during labour, including methods of assessment of fetal wellbeing.

SBA 23

Towards the end of pregnancy, the cervix becomes softer owing to the action of collagenase. Which cell type congregates in the cervix to release collagenase?

A Basophils
B Eosinophils
C Macrophages
D Neutrophils
E NK cells

Core module 11

Syllabus topic: Physiology of the third stage of labour.

SBA 24

Breastfeeding after delivery may facilitate contraction of the uterus and reduce the incidence of haemorrhage. Breastfeeding causes the release of which substance that causes uterine contraction?

A Cyclooxygenase
B Ergometrine
C Prostacyclin
D Prostaglandin F2α
E Oxytocin

Core module 12

Syllabus topic: Lactation and uterine involution.

SBA 25

Approximately how many weeks does it take for complete uterine involution following delivery?

A 1
B 2
C 6
D 12
E 24

Core module 13

Syllabus topic: Physiology of the reproductive tract in women.

SBA 26

What is considered to be the normal maximum blood loss during menstruation?

A 10 ml
B 50 ml
C 80 ml
D 120 ml
E 500 ml

Core module 14

Syllabus topics: Physiology of the reproductive tract in men and women. Regulation of gametogenesis, fertilisation and establishment of early pregnancy.

SBA 27

The glycoprotein layer surrounding a metaphase II oocyte is known as the:

A Acrosome
B Corona radiata

C Cumulus oophorus
D Polar body
E Zona pellucida

Core module 15

Syllabus topic: The impact of contraceptives on the physiology of the reproductive tract.

SBA 28
What effect does the progesterone-only pill have on the cervical mucus?

A It causes the glycoproteins to align in microscopic channels
B It causes the glycoproteins to form a dense mesh
C It causes the mucus to become thinner
D It has no effect
E It increases the water content

Core module 16

Syllabus topic: Luteoplacental shift and fetomaternal communication.

SBA 29
At what gestation does the corpus luteum cease to be essential for pregnancy maintenance?

A 4/40
B 6/40
C 12/40
D 16/40
E 20/40

Core module 17

Syllabus topic: Physiology in gynaecological oncology.

SBA 30

What percentage of women with a malignancy have hypercalcaemia?

A 1%
B 2%
C 5%
D 10%
E 20%

Core module 18

Syllabus topic: Physiology of the kidney and renal tract.

SBA 31

Where in the kidney is the majority of bicarbonate reabsorbed?

A Bowman's capsule
B Collecting duct
C Distal convoluted tubule
D Loop of Henle
E Proximal convoluted tubule

Biochemistry domain

Core modules 5–7

Syllabus topics: Structure and function of normal cells. Biochemistry of catabolism and nutrition as applied to surgery. Biochemistry of enzymes, vitamins and minerals. Effects of surgery on the fetus.

SBA 32

Which cell organelle is responsible for the enzymatic modification of secreted proteins?

A Golgi complex
B Mitochondria
C Nucleus

D Rough endoplasmic reticulum
E Smooth endoplasmic reticulum

Core module 8

Syllabus topic: Placental transfer.

SBA 33
Which fetal gland is responsible for generating dehydroepiandrosterone (DHEA) during estrogen synthesis?

A Adrenal
B Pancreas
C Parathroid
D Pituiary
E Thyroid

Core module 9

Syllabus topic: Cellular biochemistry in disorders of pregnancy.

SBA 34
Which compound inhibits hormone-sensitive lipase-mediated hydrolysis of triacylglycerol into fatty acids and glycerol?

A Adrenaline
B Gastrin
C Glucagon
D Insulin
E Noradrenaline

Core module 10

Syllabus topics: Biochemistry of prostaglandins and steroid hormones. Hormones, receptors and intracellular signalling. Biochemistry of myometrial contractility.

SBA 35

Which cellular 'second messenger' signalling molecule is generated by oxytocin stimulation of myometrial myocytes and stimulates intracellular calcium release?

A Calcium ions (Ca^{2+})
B Cyclic adenosine monophosphate (cAMP)
C Cyclic guanosine monophosphate (cGMP)
D Inositol-1,4,5,-triphosphate (IP3)
E Nitric oxide (NO)

Core module 11

Syllabus topic: Acid–base balance.

SBA 36

What type of acid–base disturbance may result from the chronic use of spironolactone (an aldosterone antagonist)?

A Metabolic acidosis
B Metabolic alkalosis
C No effect
D Respiratory acidosis
E Respiratory alkalosis

Core module 16

Syllabus topic: Hormonal changes associated with pregnancy loss.

SBA 37

A woman undergoes a surgical evacuation of retained products of conception following a miscarriage. She telephones two days later to say that her pregnancy test is still positive. What would you advise her about the length of time for which her test may remain positive? Choose the single best answer.

A 5 days
B 10 days
C 12 days

D 15 days
E 21 days

Core module 17

Syllabus topics: Regulation of the cell cycle. Cell biology in gynaecological cancer.

SBA 38
Which tumour suppressor protein is mutated in the majority of cancers?

A APC
B INK4a
C p53
D p57
E TGFβ

Embryology domain

Core modules 5–7

Syllabus topics: Developmental abnormalities in the female. Development of the urogenital tract and structural abnormalities. Structural abnormalities in the female reproductive tract.

SBA 39
Which structure in the embryo develops into the kidney and renal tract?

A Mesonephros
B Metanephros
C Müllerian duct
D Pronephros
E Wolffian duct

Core module 8

Syllabus topic: Fetal embryology.

SBA 40

The epithelium of the gastrointestinal tract develops from which germ cell layer?

A Amnion
B Ectoderm
C Endoderm
D Extraembryonic coelom
E Mesoderm

Core module 9

Syllabus topic: Fetal and placental growth and development – particularly neural tube, gut and cardiac development.

SBA 41

From which germ cell layer derivative do the autonomic ganglia develop?

A Endoderm
B Neural crest
C Neural tube
D Paraxial mesoderm
E Surface ectoderm

Core module 13

Syllabus topic: Development of the reproductive tract.

SBA 42

A bicornuate uterus is the result of the failure of which embryonic structures to correctly fuse?

A Genital tubercles
B Mesonephric ducts

C Metanephric ducts
D Paramesonephric ducts
E Pronephric ducts

Core module 14

Syllabus topics: Development of the gametes, fertilisation, implantation and early embryonic development. Regulation of the embryonic genome. Development of the reproductive tract.

SBA 43
Which embryonic cell type secretes hCG?

A Amnion
B Cytotrophoblast
C Mesoderm
D Syncytiotrophoblast
E Yolk sac

Core module 16

Syllabus topic: Chromosomal abnormalities associated with pregnancy loss.

SBA 44
What percentage of fetuses with Turner syndrome (45XO) will miscarry in the first trimester?

A 1%
B 5%
C 10%
D 50%
E 99%

Core module 18

Syllabus topic: Congenital abnormalities of the renal tract.

SBA 45

Adult polycystic kidney disease follows which pattern of inheritance?

A Autosomal dominant
B Autosomal recessive
C X-linked dominant
D X-linked recessive
E Y-linked

Epidemiology and statistics domain

Core module 1

Syllabus topics: Principles of the indications, risks, benefits and effectiveness of investigations.

SBA 46

The table below shows the results of a new test for the detection of a disease:

		Disease	
		Affected	Non-affected
Test	**Positive**	a	b
	Negative	c	d

How would you calculate the sensitivity of the new test?

A a/a+d
B a/a+c
C b/b+c
D b/b+d
E d/a+b+c

Core module 3

Syllabus topics: Principles of screening. Statistical methods used in clinical research. Principles of clinical trial design. Understand audit cycle and difference from research. Levels of evidence, quantification of risk and chance.

SBA 47

In evidence-based medicine, what level of evidence is provided by meta-analyses of randomised controlled trials?

A 1a
B 1b
C 2a
D 2b
E 3

Core module 5

Syllabus topics: Epidemiology of surgical complications. Principles of informed consent.

SBA 48

Obesity in pregnancy (BMI >30kg/m^2) increases the risk of deep vein thrombosis by approximately how many times?

A 1.2
B 2.5
C 4.4
D 14.3
E 27.1

Core module 6

Syllabus topic: Factors affecting surgical rates, operative success and complication rates.

SBA 49

A hospital appoints a new consultant with skills in endometrial ablative techniques. The management are hoping to see a decline in the overall numbers of which operation?

A Colposuspension
B Hysterectomy
C Hysteroscopy
D Laparoscopy
E Myomectomy

Core module 8

Syllabus topics: Principles of screening. Screening in pregnancy for fetal disorders. Epidemiology of disorders and complications of pregnancy. Define and interpret data on neonatal and perinatal mortality.

SBA 50

What is the World Health Organization definition of perinatal mortality?

A Number of neonatal deaths per 1000 births
B Number of stillbirths and early neonatal deaths per 1000 births
C Number of stillbirths and early neonatal deaths per 10 000 births
D Number of stillbirths per 1000 births
E Number of stillbirths per year

Core module 9

Syllabus topic: Definitions of maternal, neonatal and perinatal mortality and their interpretation.

SBA 51

What is the maternal mortality ratio?

A Ratio of number of maternal deaths and neonatal deaths
B Ratio of number of maternal deaths per 10 000 live births
C Ratio of number of maternal deaths per 100 000 live births

D Ratio of number of maternal deaths per 1 000 000 live births
E Ratio of number of maternal deaths per year per national population

Core module 13

Syllabus topic: Epidemiology of common gynaecological conditions.

SBA 52
Women from which continent are most likely to develop uterine fibroids (leiomyomata)?

A Africa
B Asia
C Australasia
D Europe
E Latin America

Core module 14

Syllabus topic: Epidemiology of infertility.

SBA 53
Which organism is responsible for the majority of cases of tubal disease leading to infertility?

A *Chlamydia trachomatis*
B Group B Streptococcus
C *Neisseria gonorrhoeae*
D *Staphylococcus aureus*
E *Treponema pallidum*

Core module 15

Syllabus topic: Epidemiology of contraception and STIs.

SBA 54
Which age group of girls is most likely to present with *Chlamydia trachomatis* infection?

A <15 years
B 15–19 years
C 20–24 years
D 25–29 years
E 30 years and above

Core module 16

Syllabus topic: Epidemiology of pregnancy failure.

SBA 55
What is the risk of miscarriage in women becoming pregnant at 45 years of age or older?

A 25%
B 37%
C 43%
D 72%
E 93%

Core module 17

Syllabus topic: Epidemiology of cancers affecting women.

SBA 56
Among women diagnosed with ovarian cancer, what is the median age at diagnosis?

A 30 years
B 38 years

C 43 years
D 55 years
E 63 years

Genetics domain

Core module 1

Syllabus topics: Structure and function of chromosomes and genes. Genomics and regulation of gene expression.

SBA 57
Nitrogenous bases make up cellular nucleic acids including DNA and RNA. Which base pairs with thymine in the standard DNA helix?

A Adenine
B Guanine
C Inosine
D Uracil
E Uranine

Core module 5

Syllabus topic: Structure and function of chromosomes and genes.

SBA 58
A normal human cell contains how many pairs of chromosomes?

A 20
B 23
C 36
D 43
E 46

Core module 7

Syllabus topic: Diagnosis of fetal anomalies.

SBA 59

What is the quoted procedure-related risk of miscarriage following amniocentesis?

A 1%
B 3%
C 5%
D 10%
E 15%

Core module 8

Syllabus topics: Chromosomal and genetic disorders – principles of inheritance. Features and effects of common inherited disorders and origins of fetal malformation.

SBA 60

What is the incidence of phenylketonuria in babies born in the UK?

A 1 in 100
B 1 in 1000
C 1 in 10 000
D 1 in 100 000
E 1 in 1 000 000

Core module 9

Syllabus topic: Genetic principles underlying screening for fetal anomaly.

SBA 61

What percentage of fetuses with trisomy 21 would be expected to be detected by a nuchal translucency scan alone (assuming a 5% false-positive rate)?

A 10%
B 25–30%
C 50–55%
D 70–75%
E 90–95%

Core module 13

Syllabus topic: Chromosome abnormalities, single gene disorders, sex-linked inheritance.

SBA 62
A fetus with Edwards' syndrome contains an extra copy of which chromosome?

A 13
B 14
C 18
D 21
E X

Core module 14

Syllabus topic: Congenital abnormalities leading to infertility.

SBA 63
A man presents to the fertility clinic with his partner. He is found to be azoospermic. He is tall and has been treated for gynaecomastia in the past. A blood sample is sent for cytogenetics. What is the most likely karyotype?

A 45XO
B 46XX
C 46XY
D 47XXX
E 47XXY

Core module 17

Syllabus topics: Genetic origins of cancer and DNA mutations. Principles of molecular testing for gynaecological cancers.

SBA 64

A woman is found to have a mutation in the BRCA1 gene. She is at increased risk of developing which cancers?

A Breast and ovarian
B Endometrial and breast
C Endometrial and colon
D Ovarian and colon
E Ovarian and endometrial

3 | Part 1 MRCOG blueprinting matrix, syllabus topics and example questions for paper 2

Answers to the questions in this chapter can be found in appendix 4.

Data interpretation domain

Core module 1

Syllabus topics: Principles of fluid and electrolyte and acid–base balance. Interpret results of investigations including microbiology swabs, haematological tests and electrolyte levels.

SBA 65

What is the most important cation in the extracellular fluid?

A Ca^{2+}
B Cl^-
C HCO_3^-
D K^+
E Na^+

Core module 3

Syllabus topic: Understand accuracy of tests used in diagnosis.

SBA 66

One hundred patients with heavy postmenopausal bleeding had a pipelle endometrial biopsy taken prior to a hysterectomy to test the ability of the biopsy to detect endometrial cancer.

		Endometrial cancer	
		Affected	Non-affected
Biopsy	Positive	20	10
	Negative	30	40

What is the specificity of the endometrial biopsy?

A 20%
B 40%
C 50%
D 80%
E 100%

Core module 5

Syllabus topic: Methods of measurement and interpretation of clinically important physiological variables as applied to surgical practice.

SBA 67

A preoperative woman with emphysema undergoes spirometry. Which lung volume is indicated by the arrows on the spirometry tracing?

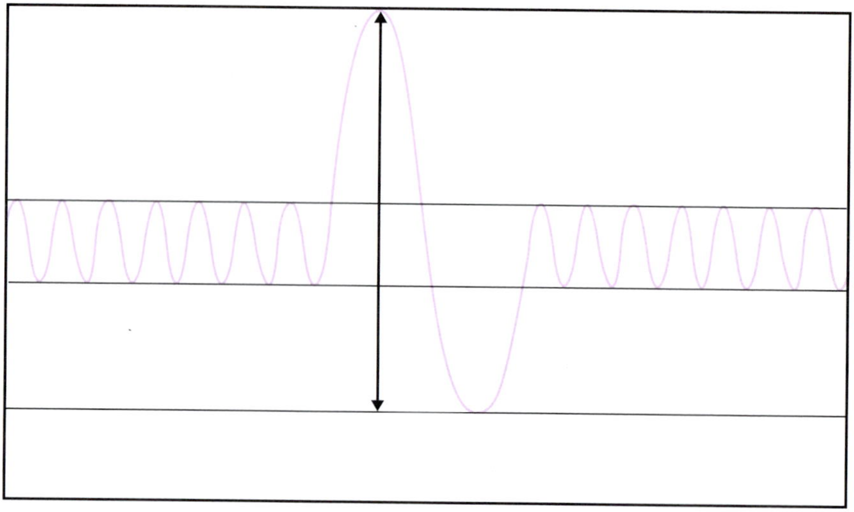

A Expiratory reserve volume
B Inspiratory reserve volume
C Tidal volume
D Total lung capacity
E Vital capacity

Core module 8

Syllabus topics: Interpret commonly performed tests in pregnancy including screening tests. Interpret data on maternal mortality.

SBA 68

An anxious 38-year-old pregnant woman undergoes a combined test for Down syndrome screening. The risk comes back as 1 in 1000. What is the appropriate course of action?

A Advise that diagnostic tests are not indicated
B Amniocentesis
C Chorionic villus sampling
D Inform the woman that the baby does not have Down syndrome
E Termination of pregnancy

Core module 9

Syllabus topics: Interpret commonly performed tests used in maternal medicine.

SBA 69

An obese, but otherwise healthy, 30-year-old woman undergoes an oral glucose tolerance test at 28 weeks of gestation. The results are as follows:

Fasting serum glucose	*5.6 mmol/l*
2-hour serum glucose	*13.5 mmol/l*

What is the diagnosis?

A Diabetic ketoacidosis
B Gestational diabetes mellitus
C Normal glucose tolerance
D Type 1 diabetes mellitus
E Type 2 diabetes mellitus

Core module 10

Syllabus topic: Interpret commonly performed tests in labour including fetal blood sampling.

SBA 70

A 27-year-old primagravida has failure to progress in the first stage of labour and is commenced on an oxytocin infusion. The midwife calls the registrar because of a suspicious CTG. The woman is found to be 6 cm dilated and the registrar performs fetal blood sampling. The sample has a pH of 7.15. What is the appropriate course of action?

A Perform an immediate caesarean section
B Perform an instrumental delivery
C Reassure the woman that all is well and the labour can continue
D Repeat the fetal blood sampling in one hour
E Repeat the fetal blood sampling in two hours

Core module 11

Syllabus topic: Interpret cord blood samples.

SBA 71

A category 1 caesarean section is undertaken for fetal distress in labour. Paired cord blood samples are taken for blood gas analysis and the results are as follows:

	Arterial	Venous
pH	7.10	7.15
Base excess	−10	−8

What type of acid–base disturbance is present?

A Metabolic acidosis
B Metabolic alkalosis
C No disturbance
D Respiratory acidosis
E Respiratory alkalosis

Core module 13

Syllabus topic: Interpret commonly performed investigations for benign gynaecological conditions.

SBA 72

A 27-year-old woman with a regular menstrual cycle is referred to the gynaecology clinic by her GP with a six-month history of intermittent right-sided abdominal pain. An ultrasound scan of the pelvis is requested and the result is as follows:

> *Day 13 of menstrual cycle. Normal uterus with endometrial thickness 13 mm. Normal left ovary. Within the right ovary is a cystic structure with dimensions 20 x 18 mm. No free fluid seen.*

What is the most likely nature of the structure in the right ovary?

A Dermoid cyst
B Endometrioma
C Mucinous cystadenoma
D Ovulatory follicle
E Serous cystadenoma

Core module 14

Syllabus topic: Interpret basic investigations for infertility.

SBA 73

A couple with secondary infertility is referred to the fertility clinic. The woman is confirmed to be ovulating and the man's semen analysis is satisfactory.

The woman undergoes a hysterosalpingogram to check her tubal patency. This is reported as follows:

> *Normal uterine cavity. Contrast is seen to enter both fallopian tubes, but there is no definite intraperitoneal spill on either side.*

What is the appropriate course of action?

A Advise to continue to try and conceive for a further year
B Diagnostic hysteroscopy
C Diagnostic laparoscopy and dye test
D Offer treatment with intrauterine insemination
E Offer treatment with in vitro fertilisation

Core module 15

Syllabus topic: Interpret results of investigations for genital tract infection.

SBA 74

A woman is referred to the genitourinary medicine clinic with a three-day history of vaginal itching, offensive vaginal discharge and dysuria. A speculum examination is performed and the cervix is noted to be inflamed. There is a moderate amount of frothy offensive discharge and swabs are sent to the laboratory. The wet film of the high vaginal swab yields a positive result. What is the most likely organism to be detected?

A *Candida albicans*
B *Chlamydia trachomatis*
C *Neisseria gonorrhoea*
D *Treponema pallidum*
E *Trichomonas vaginalis*

Core module 16

Syllabus topic: Interpret ultrasound in early pregnancy and commonly performed investigations including hCG measurement.

SBA 75

A woman attends the early pregnancy unit with heavy vaginal bleeding and crampy lower abdominal pain. It is six weeks since her last menstrual period. An ultrasound scan is performed which shows an empty uterus, normal ovaries and no free fluid in the pelvis. A serum β-hCG level is taken, which comes back at 1120 i.u./l. When the test is repeated 48 hours later, the serum β-hCG level is 580 i.u./l. What is the most likely diagnosis?

A Complete miscarriage
B Ectopic pregnancy
C Heterotopic pregnancy
D Incomplete miscarriage
E Missed miscarriage

Pathology domain

Core module 1

Syllabus topic: Understand the pathological basis of physical signs.

SBA 76

A young woman in late pregnancy presents with swelling around her ankles that indents on pressure. She is otherwise well. The single best cause for the pathological basis of this physical symptom is:

A Abnormal blood coagulation
B Fractured ankle
C Low blood pressure
D Low plasma oncotic pressure
E Low PO_2 of arterial blood

Core modules 5–7

Syllabus topic: Understand the histopathology of the pelvic organs, the breast and the endocrine organs, including the pituitary and the hypothalamus.

SBA 77

What is the single best description for the histological appearance of the endometrium soon after ovulation?

A Glands containing eosinophilic secretions with stromal breakdown and polymorphs
B Glands with subnuclear vacuolation in oedematous stroma
C Tortuous glands with cells containing high numbers of mitotic figures
D Tubular glands in compact stroma containing plasma cells
E Tubular mitotically active glands in compact stroma

Core module 8

Syllabus topics: Effect of pregnancy on disease and disease on pregnancy. Teratogenesis.

SBA 78

A woman who is 28 weeks pregnant with a fibroid uterus is admitted to the antenatal ward with severe abdominal pain. An ultrasound scan is arranged with shows a normally grown fetus and placenta, with no evidence of bleeding. Several large fibroids are noted. What is the pathological change in fibroids that can occur in pregnancy?

A Decidual degeneration
B Fibrous degeneration
C Hyaline degeneration
D Macular degeneration
E Red degeneration

Core module 11

Syllabus topic: Placental site and implantation and its abnormalities.

SBA 79

A 33-year-old woman is undergoing an elective repeat caesarean section at term. The infant is delivered without any difficulties, but the placenta cannot be removed easily because a clear plane between the placenta and uterine wall cannot be identified. The placenta is removed in pieces. What is the single most likely placental abnormality here?

A Membranaceus placenta
B Placenta accreta
C Placenta praevia
D Placental abruption
E Succenturiate lobe

Core module 13

Syllabus topics: Congenital abnormalities of the genital tract. Osteopenia/osteoporosis. Pathological conditions of the uterus (endometrium and myometrium), tubes and ovaries.

SBA 80

A 25-year-old woman presents as an emergency with severe left-sided pelvic pain and vomiting. An ultrasound scan is arranged which shows a 5 cm cystic lesion in the left adnexa with mixed echoes. A laparotomy is performed and an ovarian cyst that has undergone torsion is removed. The histology of the cyst is reported as:

> *5 cm ovary containing a cystic structure that has undergone partial necrosis. The cyst contains sebaceous material and hair. A solid element is identified that contains teeth cartilage and thyroid tissue.*

What type of cyst has torted?

A Benign cystic teratoma
B Endodermal sinus tumour
C Endometrioma
D Mucinous cystadenoma
E Serous cystadenoma

Core module 14

Syllabus topics: Pathology of tubal damage, polycystic ovary syndrome, endometriosis and the pituitary. Histology and pathology of the male genital tract.

SBA 81

A 32-year-old woman attends the fertility clinic. She has a four-year history of infertility, severe dysmenorrhoea and increasing pain with sexual intercourse. On pelvic examination, an adnexal mass is felt and nodules are palpated along the uterosacral ligaments. The single most likely cause for the pathological basis of these physical symptoms is:

A Corpus luteum cyst
B Endometriosis
C Ovarian carcinoma
D Ovarian dermoid cyst
E Pelvic inflammatory disease

Core module 15

Syllabus topics: Pathological features of STD and female genital infections. Endometrial effects of contraceptive steroids.

SBA 82

A 28-year-old woman is referred to the early pregnancy unit. She had been taking norethisterone for several weeks to delay a menstrual period while she went on holiday. She has since stopped the medication and has experienced some bleeding. She is concerned as she has passed a 'pregnancy sac' vaginally, although her pregnancy test is negative. The tissue is sent for histopathological analysis. What is the most likely diagnosis?

A Complete miscarriage
B Decidual cast
C Ectopic pregnancy
D Incomplete miscarriage
E Molar pregnancy

Core modules 16

Syllabus topic: Pathology of miscarriage, ectopic pregnancy, trophoblastic disease.

SBA 83

A 20-year-old woman is admitted to the gynaecology ward. It is six weeks since her last menstrual period and her pregnancy test is strongly positive. She is vomiting profusely and has had some vaginal bleeding. An ultrasound scan is organised and the report is as follows:

> *The uterus is very enlarged. No gestational sac is seen but the cavity is filled with tissue with a honeycombed texture. Cysts are noted on both ovaries.*

What is the most likely diagnosis?

A Choriocarcinoma
B Complete hydatidiform mole
C Endometrial carcinoma
D Endometrial hyperplasia
E Partial hydatidiform mole

Core module 17

Syllabus topics: Pathology, histology and classification of gynaecological cancers and premalignant conditions. Field change effects. Aetiological factors. Cervical cytology. Pathology of pain and transmission of pain signals centrally.

SBA 84

Which two HPV types are found in 70% of cervical cancers and are targeted in HPV vaccines?

A 6 and 11
B 16 and 18
C 31 and 35
D 31 and 45
E 73 and 82

Core module 18

Syllabus topic: Pathological conditions of the bladder, urethra and vagina.

SBA 85

What type of epithelial tissue undergoes malignant change in the majority of bladder cancers?

A Columnar
B Pseudostratified
C Squamous
D Stratified
E Transitional

Pharmacology domain

Core module 1

Syllabus topic: Safe prescribing, avoiding drug errors, drug interactions, adverse effects.

SBA 86

A woman who has been taking the combined oral contraceptive pill for many years is commenced on phenytoin following a seizure. She then becomes pregnant. Through what mechanism is the contraceptive pill likely to have failed?

A Alteration of gut flora by phenytoin
B Antagonistic effects of phenytoin at the estrogen receptor
C Increased renal clearance of the contraceptive pill
D Liver enzyme induction by phenytoin
E Liver enzyme inhibition by phenytoin

Core module 3

Syllabus topic: Comparison of effectiveness/cost-effectiveness, number needed to treat.

SBA 87

For an ideal drug, where everyone improves with treatment and no-one improves with placebo, what is the number needed to treat?

A 1
B 2
C 5
D 10
E 100

Core module 5

Syllabus topic: Pharmacokinetics and factors affecting drug action.

SBA 88

Renal clearance of most drugs is altered in pregnancy. In the table below, which option correctly identifies the normal physiological changes in pregnancy that have an impact on pharmacokinetics?

	Circulating volume	Renal blood flow	Serum albumin
A	Increased	Decreased	Decreased
B	Increased	Increased	Decreased
C	Decreased	Increased	Decreased
D	Decreased	Decreased	Increased
E	Increased	Increased	Increased

Core module 6

Syllabus topics: Properties and actions of drugs used after surgery. Antibiotics and antibiotic prophylaxis.

SBA 89

To reduce surgical-site infections, prophylactic antibiotics are often used. When is the ideal time to administer such prophylaxis?

A Six hours before surgery
B Three hours before surgery
C At induction of anaesthesia
D Four hours after surgery
E Six hours after surgery

Core module 7

Syllabus topics: Properties and actions of drugs, including anaesthetic agents used during surgery. Effect of drugs on haemostasis and uterine bleeding.

SBA 90

What is the most common drug used for induction of anaesthesia in non-obstetric patients in the UK?

A Halothane
B Lidocaine
C Propofol
D Suxamethonium
E Thiopentone

Core module 8

Syllabus topics: Prescribing in pregnancy. Placental handling of drugs. Effects of drugs on the pregnant woman and fetus. Drugs for fetal development and wellbeing.

SBA 91

A woman is admitted with threatened preterm labour. Two doses of corticosteroids are administered to promote fetal lung maturity. Over what time period after the second dose are the corticosteroids most effective in reducing respiratory distress syndrome if delivery occurs?

A 10–15 hours
B 18–24 hours
C 24 hours to 7 days
D 7–10 days
E 10–14 days

Core module 9

Syllabus topics: Drugs and their adverse effects in pregnancy. Drugs used in pregnancy-specific pathologies and complications of pregnancy.

SBA 92

A 28-year-old asthmatic woman develops pre-eclampsia at 34 weeks of gestation and a decision is made to commence antihypertensive therapy. She has previously experienced adverse effects with nifedipine and wishes to avoid this drug. Which antihypertensive agent will be suitable for her?

A Atenolol
B Bendroflumethazide
C Labetalol
D Lisinopril
E Methyldopa

Core module 10

Syllabus topics: Tocolysis and stimulants of uterine contractility. Pain relief in labour and the puerperium.

SBA 93

A woman is admitted with threatened preterm labour and is commenced on atosiban. What is the mechanism of action of atosiban?

A Calcium channel blocker
B GnRH analogue
C GnRH antagonist
D Oxytocin agonist
E Oxytocin antagonist

Core module 11

Syllabus topics: Drugs in management of delivery. Third stage of labour and its problems. Effects of drugs on the newborn.

SBA 94

A woman experiences a postpartum haemorrhage after delivery and is administered ergometrine to promote uterine contraction. What class of compound is ergometrine?

A Alkaloid
B Eicosanoid
C Polypepetide
D Protein
E Steroid

Core module 12

Syllabus topics: Contraception in the postpartum period. Use of drugs during lactation.

SBA 95

Cabergoline may be used to suppress lactation in women who have suffered a stillbirth. Through which mechanism of action and which receptor does cabergonline suppress lactation?

A Agonist at β receptor
B Agonist at D1 receptor
C Agonist at D2 receptor
D Antagonist at D1 receptor
E Antagonist at D2 receptor

Core module 13

Syllabus topic: Drugs in benign gynaecology, including treatment of menorrhagia, dysmenorrhoea, endometriosis, polycystic ovary syndrome, menopause, osteoporosis.

SBA 96

Tranexamic acid is a first-line treatment for menorrhagia. What is the mechanism of action of tranexamic acid?

A Antifibrinolytic
B Cyclooxygenase inhibitor
C GnRH analogue
D Oxytocin antagonist
E Progestogen

Core module 14

Syllabus topics: Drugs used to treat infertilty. Drugs used in anovulation, superovulation and assisted conception. Drug teratogenicity. Drugs that interfere with fertility.

SBA 97

Clomifene is a commonly used drug for the induction of ovulation. By which mechanism does clomifene promote follicular development?

A Binds to estrogen receptors in the endometrium
B Binds to estrogen receptors in the pituitary, promoting an LH surge
C Blocks estrogen receptors in the hypothalamus, increasing FSH pulse frequency
D Increases inhibin production by the ovary
E Opposes ovarian anti-müllerian hormone production

Core module 15

Syllabus topics: Contraceptives. Drugs used for medical termination of pregnancy. Drugs used for STIs, including antimicrobial resistance.

SBA 98

Mifepristone is a drug used in the medical termination of pregnancy. What is mifepristone's mode of action?

A Estrogen agonist
B Estrogen antagonist
C Oxytocin antagonist
D Progesterone agonist
E Progesterone antagonist

Core module 16

Syllabus topic: Medical management of miscarriage, trophoblastic disease and ectopic pregnancy.

SBA 99

Misoprostol is a commonly used drug in the medical management of miscarriage. What type of drug is misoprostol?

A Cyclooxygenase inhibitor
B Oxytocin antagonist
C Progesterone antagonist
D Progestogen
E Synthetic prostaglandin

Core module 17

Syllabus topics: Properties and actions of drugs used to treat gynaecological cancers and trophoblastic disorders. Effects of chemotherapeutic agents on gonadal function.

SBA 100

Some women who have gestational trophoblastic disease require chemotherapy, either with methotrexate or with a combination of drugs. How long should such women wait to try and conceive after they have completed their chemotherapy treatment?

A One month
B Two months
C Three months
D Six months
E 12 months

Core module 18

Syllabus topic: Properties and actions of drugs used in urogynaecology.

SBA 101

A 75-year-old woman attends the gynaecology clinic. She has been receiving medical treatment for overactive bladder for many years, but her notes are not available today and she has forgotten to bring the medication with her. On questioning, she reveals that the medication gives her a terrible dry mouth, dry eyes, blurred vision and constipation. Which drug is she most likely to be taking?

A Duloxetine
B Oxybutynin
C Phenoxybenzamine
D Sertraline
E Sibutramine

Biophysics domain

Core module 5

Syllabus topics: Principles of electrocardiography, ultrasound, Doppler, X-rays and MRI. Use of laser and electrosurgery.

SBA 102
The QRS complex in a normal electrocardiogram represents:

A Atrial depolarisation and contraction
B The electrical activity of the sinoatrial node
C The final stage of ventricular repolarisation
D Ventricular depolarisation and contraction
E Ventricular repolarisation

Core module 9

Syllabus topic: Physics of Doppler, ultrasound and magnetic resonance imaging.

SBA 103
The lateral resolution of an ultrasound image/system depends on:

A The acoustic power
B The frequency
C The position of the focus
D The slice thickness
E The type of transducer used

Core module 14

Syllabus topics: Use of transvaginal and transabdominal ultrasound. X-ray and hysterosalpingography.

SBA 104

X-rays have frequencies in the range:

A 2×10^3 Hz to 2×10^4 Hz
B 1×10^6 Hz to 20×10^6 Hz
C 5×10^{10} Hz to 5×10^{11} Hz
D 4×10^{14} Hz to 8×10^{14} Hz
E 5×10^{18} Hz to 50×10^{18} Hz

Core module 16

Syllabus topic: Ultrasound in early pregnancy.

SBA 105

At what serum hCG level should an experienced sonographer using transvaginal ultrasonography expect to detect an intrauterine gestational sac in a normally developing pregnancy?

A 10
B 50
C 100
D 500
E 1000

Core module 17

Syllabus topics: Physics of laser and MRI. Principles of radiotherapy.

SBA 106

Magnetic resonance imaging uses the following physical principle to form an image:

A Acceleration of electrons
B Conversion of low-frequency current to high-frequency current
C Stimulated emission of radiation
D The alignment of protons in water
E Vibration of a piezo-electric crystal

Core module 18

Syllabus topic: Principles of measurement of bladder function.

SBA 107

What is the main muscle being evaluated during urodynamic testing?

A Detrusor
B Levator ani
C Pyramidalis
D Pyriformis
E Rectus abdominis

Clinical management domain

Core module 1

Syllabus topics: Analyse an obstetric and gynaecological history. Understand the principles underpinning clinical examinations. Aware of Fraser competence issues.

SBA 108

The Fraser guidelines require doctors to be satisfied that certain criteria are met before offering treatment to minors under 16 years of age without parental consent. To which type of treatment do they specifically refer?

A Abortion
B Antibiotic treatment
C Contraception
D Sexually transmitted infections
E Surgery

Core module 5

Syllabus topics: Demonstrate knowledge of the principles underpinning fluid and electrolyte balance, and coagulation. Demonstrate knowledge of the basic clinical skills in core surgical practice.

SBA 109

Following a routine hysterectomy, a woman is prescribed intravenous fluids. Unfortunately, an infusion pump is not available and the fluid-giving set is incorrectly set up, resulting in the woman receiving six litres of fluid in 24 hours. The following day on the ward round she is noted to be breathless with low oxygen saturation. What is the most likely complication she has suffered?

A Acute respiratory distress syndrome
B Bronchitis
C Deep venous thrombosis
D Pulmonary embolus
E Pulmonary oedema

Core module 6

Syllabus topic: Show understanding of the management surrounding surgical complications, infection and infection control.

SBA 110

Regarding laparoscopic entry technique, which type of injury is likely to be reduced by the open (Hasson) technique as opposed to the closed (Veress needle) technique?

A Bladder injury
B Large bowel injury
C Major vessel injury
D Small bowel injury
E Uterine injury

Core module 7

Syllabus topic: Principles of procedures used in surgical practice.

SBA 111

What is the risk of uterine perforation at hysteroscopy?

A 0.01%
B 0.1%
C 1%
D 10%
E 15%

Core module 8

Syllabus topic: Principles underlying the management of common disorders of pregnancy.

SBA 112

A woman who is 11 weeks pregnant is referred to the gynaecology ward with a two-week history of vomiting. She is prescribed intravenous rehydration and anti-emetics. She should also be prescribed which vitamin to reduce the chance of Wernicke's encephalopathy?

A Vitamin A
B Vitamin B_1
C Vitamin B_6
D Vitamin B_{12}
E Vitamin C

Core module 9

Syllabus topic: Principles underlying the management of common disorders of pregnancy complicated by maternal disease.

SBA 113

A 25-year-old primagravida presents at 34 weeks of pregnancy with intense itching, which is worse on the palms of her hands and soles of her feet. A set of liver function tests is requested, with the following results:

Albumin	29 g/l	(35–50)
Serum alkaline phosphatase	279 u/l	(40–120)
Alanine transaminase	80 u/l	(0–45)
Gamma GT	50 u/l	(0–45)
Bilirubin	19 μmol/l	(0–21)

What other blood test would you request at this stage?

A Bile acids
B Calcium and phosphate levels
C Full blood count
D Urea and electrolytes
E Viral hepatitis screen

Core module 10

Syllabus topic: Understand the principles of management of labour.

SBA 114

A midwife calls the obstetric registrar to review a labouring woman. The partogram shows no progress of cervical dilatation for the past four hours. The cervix is currently 7 cm dilated and the membranes are intact. The midwife is also concerned that the CTG is suspicious. What is the next course of action?

A Advise the woman to mobilise and review again in two hours
B Arrange a caesarean section
C Commence an oxytocin infusion
D Perform artificial rupture of membranes
E Perform fetal blood sampling

Core module 11

Syllabus topic: Understand the principles of operative delivery and perineal repair.

SBA 115

Following a forceps delivery, a woman is found to have extensive vaginal and perineal tears. When she is examined in theatre by the obstetric registrar, it is noted that approximately 40% of the external anal sphincter is torn, although the internal anal sphincter is intact. What degree of tear is this?

A 2
B 3a
C 3b
D 3c
E 4

Core module 12

Syllabus topic: Understand the principles of management of post-partum problems, including haemorrhage.

SBA 116

Following a water birth, a woman elects not to have oxytocics for the management of the third stage of labour. Thirty minutes later, she is brought to the consultant unit with a postpartum haemorrhage owing to an atonic uterus. If she had received standard oxytocic management for the third stage of labour, by what amount would she have reduced her risk of a postpartum haemorrhage?

A 10%
B 20%
C 30%
D 60%
E 90%

Core module 13

Syllabus topic: Understand the principles of management of common gynaecological problems.

SBA 117

An overweight 80-year-old woman with type 2 diabetes mellitus and atrial fibrillation is referred to the gynaecology clinic with a 'lump down below' which is troubling her. She is examined by the registrar, who finds a moderate-sized cystocele but no rectocele. What would be the most appropriate first-line management?

A Insertion of a ring pessary
B Insertion of a shelf pessary
C Physiotherapy referral
D Treatment with hormone replacement therapy
E Vaginal hysterectomy and pelvic floor repair

Core module 14

Syllabus topic: Understand the principles of management of subfertility.

SBA 118

A 45-year-old woman who is fit and well is referred to the fertility clinic as she would like to become pregnant. She has marked oligomenorrhoea. Basic tests are organised for the woman and her husband with the following results:

FSH: 22.3 i.u./l (1–11 i.u./l)
Progesterone (mid-luteal): <2 nmol/l (>30 nmol/l)
Ultrasound: Normal uterus. Ovaries not clearly seen.
Hysterosalpingogram: Normal uterine cavity. Both tubes patent.
Semen analysis × 2: Normal

What treatment will give them the greatest chance of achieving a pregnancy?

A Clomifene citrate
B Intrauterine insemination
C IVF
D IVF with donor eggs
E IVF with donor sperm

Core module 15

Syllabus topics: Understand the principles of management of STD. Understand the prescribing of contraception.

SBA 119

A 21-year-old woman with a new sexual partner attends the Accident and Emergency department with fever, lower abdominal pain and vaginal discharge. She is otherwise well. She is examined and appropriate swabs are taken. A pregnancy test is negative and an ultrasound scan is organised which is unremarkable. What is the appropriate course of action?

A Admit to hospital for intravenous antibiotics
B Arrange a laparoscopy
C Arrange a laparotomy
D Commence treatment with antibiotics and manage as an outpatient
E Discharge home and wait for the results of the swabs

Core module 16

Syllabus topic: Understand the principles of management of early pregnancy failure.

SBA 120

Following early pregnancy loss, women can be offered expectant, medical or surgical management. What percentage of women express a strong preference for surgical evacuation of the uterus?

A 12%
B 19%
C 34%
D 64%
E 82%

Core module 17

Syllabus topic: Understand the principles of management of gynaecological cancer.

SBA 121

An 80-year-old woman is admitted to the gynaecology ward with heavy postmenopausal bleeding. A hysteroscopy and endometrial biopsy are performed and the histology result confirms an endometrial carcinoma. What is the most appropriate next step?

A Arrange an abdominal hysterectomy
B Arrange a vaginal hysterectomy
C Refer for radiotherapy
D Refer the case to the multidisciplinary team meeting for a management plan
E Refer to palliative care

Core module 18

Syllabus topic: Understand the principles of management of disorders of the urinary tract and perineum.

SBA 122

A 60-year-old woman is referred to the gynaecology clinic with symptoms of urinary urgency and frequency, nocturia and urge incontinence. She also leaks urine when coughing or sneezing. Physical examination is unremarkable, with no evidence of pelvic floor prolapse, and a mid-stream urine sample is clear. What is the most appropriate course of action?

A Arrange a laparoscopic colposuspension
B Arrange an anterior repair
C Arrange insertion of a tension-free vaginal tape
D Arrange urodynamic testing
E Commence treatment with oxybutynin

Immunology domain

Core modules 5–7

Syllabus topics: Organisation of immune system. Immunogenetics and principles of antigen recognition. Immunology of graft rejection and immune responses in infection, inflammation and trauma.

SBA 123

Which immunoglobulin class has a pentameric structure and is unable to cross the placenta?

A IgA
B IgD
C IgE
D IgG
E IgM

Core module 8

Syllabus topic: Maternofetal immunology.

SBA 124

What is the immunological basis of haemolytic disease of the newborn (rhesus disease) and the correct associated therapy?

A RhD-negative mother carries RhD-negative fetus: administer D^+ serum
B RhD-negative mother carries RhD-positive fetus: administer anti-D serum
C RhD-positive mother carries Rh-negative fetus: administer D^+ serum
D RhD-positive mother carries RhD-positive fetus: administer anti-D serum
E RhD-positive mother, RhD-positive father: administer anti-D serum

Core module 9

Syllabus topics: Immunology of pregnancy. The fetus as an allograft. Isoimmunisation.

SBA 125

The pregnant uterus is viewed as immune privileged. What is the cellular basis for this phenomenon?

A Extravillous trophoblasts do not express higher levels of the MHC-1 antigens HLA-A and HLA-B but do express HLA-E and HLA-G
B Extravillous trophoblasts express higher levels of the highly polymorphic MHC-1 antigen HLA-G
C Extravillous trophoblasts express higher levels of the MHC-1 antigens HLA-A, HLA-B, HLA-C and HLA-G
D Syncytiotrophoblasts do not express higher levels of the MHC-1 antigens HLA-A and HLA-B but do express HLA-C and HLA-G
E Syncytiotrophoblasts express higher levels of the MHC-1 antigens HLA-A, HLA-B, HLA-E and HLA-G

Core module 13

Syllabus topics: Immunology of tissue grafting and graft rejection. Immune responses to infection, inflammation and trauma. Graft-versus-host reaction, autoimmunity, immunisation and immunosuppression.

SBA 126

What type of immune hypersensitivity reaction best describes haemolytic disease of the newborn (rhesus disease)?

A Type I (immediate) hypersensitivity
B Type II (antibody-mediated) hypersensitivity
C Type III (immune-complex) hypersensitivity
D Type IV (delayed-type) hypersensitivity
E Type V (suppressive-type) hypersensitivity

Core module 14

Syllabus topic: Principles of reproductive immunology.

SBA 127

Naive CD4-positive T cells can polarise to become either Th1 or Th2 phenotypes depending upon the nature of the signals they receive. What is the balance between Th1 and Th2 cells during pregnancy and which signal is involved?

A Th1 activated: Th2 suppressed; IFN-γ neutral
B Th1 suppressed: Th2 increased; IFN-γ predominates
C Th1 suppressed: Th2 increased; IFN-γ suppressed
D Th1:Th2 levels are the same; IFN-γ predominates
E Th1:Th2 levels are the same; IFN-γ suppressed

Core module 16

Syllabus topic: Immunology of pregnancy and miscarriage.

SBA 128

The conversion of prothrombin to thrombin can be inhibited by lupus anticoagulant antibodies. What is the frequency of these antibodies in the normal UK obstetric population and the risk of fetal mortality associated with such antisera?

A 0.5–1% of normal population; 70–75% risk of fetal mortality
B 1–2% of normal population; 70–80% risk of fetal mortality
C 2–5% of normal population; 85–95% risk of fetal mortality
D 1–2% of normal population; 75–80% risk of fetal mortality
E 2–5% of normal population; 75–80% risk of fetal mortality

Core module 17

Syllabus topic: Tumour surveillance and immunotherapy.

SBA 129

Biochemical markers can be used to indicate the presence of a tumour. Which serum marker is used to screen for trophoblastic tumours?

A Activin-A
B α-FP
C BRCA1
D CA125
E hCG

Microbiology domain

Core modules 5–7

Syllabus topics: Biology of microorganisms encountered in surgical practice. Principles of infection control. Principles of antimicrobial prophylaxis and wound care.

SBA 130

It is estimated that surgical-site infections account for 9% of all hospital-acquired infections. Which bacteria are most commonly associated with such infections?

A *Candida albicans*
B *Cryptococcus neoformans*
C *Plasmodium falciparum*
D *Staphylococcus aureus*
E *Trichomonas vaginalis*

Core module 8

Syllabus topics: Infection in pregnancy. Screening for infection. Virus biology.

SBA 131

Roughly 60% of babies born to mothers who carry group B Streptococcus (GBS) will also become colonised as they pass through the vagina at birth. Which strain of Streptococcus is responsible for the majority of GBS infections?

A *Streptococcus agalactiae*
B *Streptococcus angiosus*
C *Streptococcus bovis*
D *Streptococcus pneumoniae*
E *Streptococcus pyogenes*

Core module 9

Syllabus topics: Infectious complications of pregnancy and their management. Fetal impact of maternal infection.

SBA 132

Ascending infection of the vagina can induce premature labour. Which pathogen is most commonly associated with bacterial vaginosis?

A *Candida albicans*
B *Chlamyidia trachomatis*
C *Gardnerella vaginalis*
D *Listeria monocytogenes*
E *Neisseria meningitidis*

Core modules 10–11

Syllabus topic: Infection and its management in labour and delivery.

SBA 133

In the UK obstetric population, a risk-based approach is employed to determine which women will benefit from prophylactic antibiotic treatment for group B Streptococcus infection. Assuming the woman does not have an allergy to penicillin-based antibiotics, which antibiotic is used for prophylaxis during labour?

A Ampicillin
B Benzylpenicillin
C Cefalexin
D Clindamycin
E Flucloxacillin

Core module 12

Syllabus topics: Puerperal sepsis. Infection and its management in the postpartum period.

SBA 134

A woman who had prolonged rupture of membranes presents to hospital three days after a spontaneous vaginal delivery with abdominal pain, fever and vaginal bleeding. On examination the uterus is tender. The cervix is closed but bleeding is noted with an offensive odour. What is the most likely diagnosis?

A Endometriosis
B Endometritis
C Pelvic inflammatory disease
D Retained products of conception
E Urinary tract infection

Core module 13

Syllabus topic: Infectious diseases in gynaecological practice.

SBA 135

A woman presents to the Accident and Emergency department with a painful swelling on the left side of the vaginal introitus. She was recently treated for pelvic inflammatory disease. Which gland is most likely to be infected?

A Bartholin's gland
B Nabothian gland
C Sebaceous gland
D Skene's gland
E Sweat gland

Core module 14

Syllabus topic: Pelvic inflammatory disease and its effects on fertility.

SBA 136

Which organism causes tubal infection that is responsible for the majority of cases of secondary infertility?

A *Chlamydia trachomatis*
B *Mycobacterium tuberculosis*
C *Neisseria gonorrhoeae*
D *Treponema pallidum pallidum*
E *Treponema pallidum pertenue*

Core module 15

Syllabus topic: Sexually transmitted infections.

SBA 137

Which pathogen underlies late congenital infection during childhood and presents with eighth-nerve deafness, interstitial keratitis and abnormal teeth?

A *Chlamydia trachomatis*
B *Mycobacterium tuberculosis*
C *Neisseria gonorrhoeae*
D *Treponema pallidum pallidum*
E *Treponema pallidum pertenue*

Core module 16

Syllabus topic: Infective factors predisposing to pregnancy loss and ectopic pregnancy.

SBA 138

Chorioamnionitis infections increase the risk of preterm birth by two- to three-fold. What is the azithromycin-sensitive pathogen which can cause chorioamnionitis?

A *Chlamydia trachomatis*
B *Clostridium botulinum*
C *Listeria monocytogenes*
D *Streptococcus mutans*
E *Vibrio cholerae*

Core module 17

Syllabus topic: HPV and other viral origins of cancer.

SBA 139

HPV-16 and HPV-18 are the most common high-risk types of infection leading to cervical cancer. What are the key cellular proteins targeted by HPV E6 and E7 proteins?

A A20 and IκBα
B Cyclin E and cyclin-dependant kinase-4
C Helicase and telomerase
D NF-κB and p300
E p53 and pRb

Core module 18

Syllabus topic: Urinary tract infection.

SBA 140

Which organism is implicated in the majority of urinary tract infections in pregnancy?

A *Escherichia coli*
B Group B Streptococcus
C *Pseudomonas aeruginosa*
D *Staphylococcus aureus*
E *Trichomonas vaginalis*

4 | Mock paper: paper 1

Answers to the questions in this chapter can be found in appendix 5.

1 From which germ cell layer are the ureters derived?

A Ectoderm
B Endoderm
C Mesoderm
D Trophoblast
E Yolk sac

2 The urachus becomes fibrosed and obliterated to form which structure in the adult?

A Falciform ligament
B Lateral umbilical ligament
C Ligamentum teres
D Medial umbilical ligament
E Median umbilical ligament

3 A pudendal nerve block is used in obstetrics to provide analgesia for instrumental delivery. The pudendal nerve derives fibres from which spinal segments?

A L4–5
B L5, S1
C S2–4
D S3–5
E S4–5

4 Which structure is attached to the lateral aspect of the cervix and the lateral wall of the pelvis and is one of the main supports of the uterus?

A Broad ligament
B Ovarian ligament
C Round ligament
D Transverse cervical ligament
E Uterosacral ligament

5 The majority of the lymphatic drainage of the breast passes to which group of lymph nodes?

A Axillary nodes
B Inguinal nodes
C Para-aortic nodes
D Superficial cervical nodes
E Supraclavicular nodes

6 How many tendinous intersections are there in each rectus abdominis muscle?

A 1
B 2
C 3
D 4
E 5

7 The inferior epigastric artery is a branch of which artery?

A External iliac artery
B Femoral artery
C Internal iliac artery
D Umbilical artery
E Uterine artery

8 Which muscles form the pelvic floor?

A Levator ani and coccygeus
B Levator ani and piriformis
C Obturator internus and coccygeus
D Obturator internus and levator ani
E Obturator internus and piriformis

9 Which muscles are contained in the deep perineal pouch?

A Deep transverse perineal muscles and bulbospongiosus
B Deep transverse perineal muscles and the urethral sphincter
C Ischiocavernosus and bulbospongiosus
D Superficial transverse perineal muscles and bulbospongiosus
E Superficial transverse perineal muscles and the urethral sphincter

10 Which nerve supplies the external anal sphincter?

A Femoral nerve
B Ilioinguinal nerve
C Inferior rectal nerve
D Pelvic splanchnic nerves
E Superior rectal nerve

11 The infundibulopelvic ligament contains which artery?

A External iliac artery
B Internal iliac artery
C Inferior mesenteric artery
D Ovarian artery
E Uterine artery

12 The internal pudendal artery is a branch of which artery?

A Inferior gluteal artery
B Inferior rectal artery
C Internal iliac artery
D Superior mesenteric artery
E Umbilical artery

13

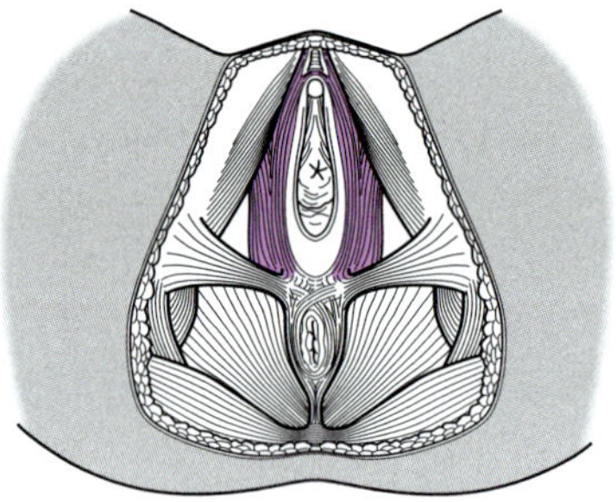

Which muscle is indicated in purple in the above diagram?

A Bulbospongiosus
B Deep transverse perineal muscles
C External anal sphincter
D Ischiocavernosus
E Superficial transverse perineal muscles

14 At laparoscopy, the obliterated umbilical artery can be seen in the adult. This structure is known as:

A Falciform ligament
B Lateral umbilical ligament
C Ligamentum teres
D Medial umbilical ligament
E Median umbilical ligament

15 Which key cellular 'second messenger' signalling molecule is generated from the precursor amino acid L-arginine?

A Calcium ions
B Cyclic adenosine monophosphate (cAMP)
C Cyclic guanosine monophosphate (cGMP)
D Inositol 1,4,5,-trisphosphate
E Nitric oxide (NO)

16 Which essential molecule in cellular metabolism helps promote iron absorption from the gastrointestinal system?

A Acetyl coenzyme A
B Lactic acid
C L-ascorbic acid
D Glucose
E Glucuronic acid

17 Aspirin and other NSAIDs are often contraindicated in individuals with asthma. The activity of which enzyme can exacerbate airway inflammation in such individuals?

A Carbonic anhydrase
B Cyclooxygenase 2
C Hormone-sensitive lipase
D Lipoxygenase
E UDP-glucuronyl transferase

18 In the absence of oxygen, cells rely on anaerobic metabolism to satisfy their need for ATP. What are the biochemical changes associated with prolonged anaerobic respiration?

A Decreased lactate levels; serum pH decreased
B Decreased lactate levels; serum pH elevated
C Increased lactate levels; serum pH decreased
D Increased lactate levels; serum pH elevated
E Increased plasma free fatty acid levels; serum pH unchanged

19 Human plasma has a pH in the range of 7.35–7.45. One element that maintains this pH is the bicarbonate buffer system. What is the normal human plasma bicarbonate (HCO_3^-) concentration?

A 8–11 mmol/l
B 12–18 mmol/l
C 19–22 mmol/l
D 23–28 mmol/l
E 29–33 mmol/l

20 Primordial germ cells originate in which structure in the embryo?

A Amniotic cavity
B Genital ridge
C Paramesonephric duct
D Pronephros
E Yolk sac

21 From which embryonic structure does the penis develop in the male?

A Genital fold
B Genital swelling
C Genital tubercle
D Paramesonephric duct
E Urogenital sinus

22 The renal tubules of the kidney develop from which embryonic tissue?

A Endoderm
B Mesonephros
C Metanephric mesoderm
D Pronephros
E Ureteric bud

23 A person has been diagnosed as having androgen insensitivity syndrome (AIS). What is the correct genotype and phenotype?

	Genotype	Phenotype
A	46XY	Female
B	46XY	Male
C	46XX	Female
D	46XX	Male
E	46XO	Female

24 Derivatives of the primitive midgut in the adult are supplied by which artery?

A Coeliac trunk
B Common iliac artery
C Femoral artery
D Inferior mesenteric artery
E Superior mesenteric artery

25 What type of compound is human placental lactogen?

A Carbohydrate
B Fatty acid
C Prostaglandin
D Protein
E Steroid

26 In the adult, growth hormone affects growth, metabolism and cell differentiation. Where, in the pituitary gland, are the cells that secrete growth hormone?

A Infundibulum
B Median eminence
C Pars distalis
D Pars nervosa
E Pars tuberalis

27 Which pituitary hormone in the non-pregnant adult is structurally most similar to prolactin?

A FSH
B GnRH
C Growth hormone
D LH
E TSH

28 In normal puberty in girls, which physical change appears first?

A Axillary hair growth
B Breast development
C Menstruation
D Pubic hair growth
E Skin changes, e.g. acne

29 A previously fit woman presents to the endocrine clinic with enlarged hands and feet, jaw protrusion, arthralgia and excessive sweating. What is the most likely diagnosis?

A Acromegaly
B Addison's disease
C Cushing's disease
D Graves' disease
E Hyperprolactinaemia

30 Two months after a normal delivery complicated by a large postpartum haemorrhage, a woman presents with failure of lactation, amenorrhoea, tiredness and loss of pubic hair. What is the most likely diagnosis?

A Cushing syndrome
B Diabetes mellitus
C Premature ovarian failure
D Prolactinoma
E Sheehan syndrome

31 Which hormone is deficient in people with diabetes insipidus?

A Arginine vasopressin
B Growth hormone
C Insulin
D Insulin-like growth factor
E Oxytocin

32 Which steroid hormone accounts for approximately 90% of mineralocorticoid activity in the body?

A 17-hydroxyprogesterone
B Aldosterone
C Corticosterone
D Cortisol
E Pregnenolone

33 A 40-year-old woman presents to the endocrine clinic with anxiety, palpitations, sweating and weakness. She has an obvious goitre. What is the most likely cause of her hyperthyroidism?

A Graves' disease
B Thyroid follicular carcinoma
C Thyroiditis
D Toxic adenoma
E Toxic multinodular goitre

34 Which cell type, in the islets of Langerhans, secretes glucagon?

A Alpha cells
B Beta cells
C Delta cells
D Epsilon cells
E PP cells

35 What statistical value provides details of how close a sample mean is to the population mean?

A Coefficient of variation
B Confidence interval
C Standard deviation
D Standard error of the mean
E Variance around the mean

36 The null hypothesis states that a given variable is without effect. What type of error is present when the null hypothesis is incorrectly not rejected?

A Alpha or type I error
B Beta or type II error
C Delta or type III error
D Gamma or type IV error
E Omega or type V error

37 What is the best description of the power of a study?

A The study's ability to correct for sampling errors
B The study's ability to detect an effect around the mean
C The study's ability to detect an effect of a specified size
D The study's ability to detect differences in the mean
E The study's ability to predict confidence limits

38 Concerning the epidemiology of maternal mortality, what is the definition of coincidental maternal death?

A Direct deaths per 100 000 live births
B Direct deaths per 100 000 maternities
C Indirect deaths per 100 000 live births
D Maternal deaths resulting from causes unrelated to pregnancy
E Maternal deaths resulting from complications unique to pregnancy

39 A woman presents to the maternity unit with no fetal movements at 22 weeks of gestation. An ultrasound scan is performed, which shows that the fetus has died in utero. What is the correct epidemiological term related to fetal and neonatal deaths to describe this phenomenon?

A Early fetal loss
B Early neonatal death
C Late fetal loss
D Late neonatal death
E Stillbirth

40 Probability is the measure of a given observation occurring by chance and is denoted by the symbol P. What value of P indicates that an observation will definitely occur?

A $P = 1$
B $P = 0.5$
C $P = 0.1$
D $P = 0.01$
E $P = 0.001$

41 A new antenatal screening test to assess the level of cervical effacement in threatened preterm delivery has been developed. In trials this test has a high degree of specificity. What is the definition of the term 'specificity'?

A The proportion of false positives that is correctly identified by the test
B The proportion of people with negative results who are correctly diagnosed by the test
C The proportion of people with positive results who are correctly diagnosed by the test
D The proportion of true negatives that is correctly identified by the test
E The proportion of true positives that is correctly identified by the test

42 What is the name of the syndrome characterised by trisomy at chromosome 13?

A Down syndrome
B Edwards' syndrome
C Klinefelter syndrome
D Lorain–Levi syndrome
E Patau syndrome

43 Nitrogenous bases make up cellular nucleic acids including DNA and RNA. Which base forms hydrogen bonds with cytosine in the DNA double helix?

A Adenine
B Guanine
C Inosine
D Uracil
E Uranine

44 What is the name of the chromosome rearrangement that involves the transfer of genetic material between two non-homologous chromosomes?

A Frameshift mutation
B Nonsense mutation
C Reciprocal translocation
D Robertsonian translocation
E Triplet repeat expansion

45 Which genetic microdeletion at loci 4p15 gives the affected individual a facial appearance with 'Greek helmet' profile?

A Cri du chat syndrome
B Langer–Giedion syndrome
C Smith–Magenis syndrome
D Williams syndrome
E Wolf–Hirschhorn syndrome

46 Cystic fibrosis is an autosomal recessive genetic condition which affects the *CFTR* gene. If both parents are heterozygous for the *CFTR* mutation, what is the probability of them having an affected child?

A One in two
B One in four
C One in eight
D One in 16
E One in 32

47 Achondroplasia is an autosomal dominant genetic condition which affects the *FGF3* gene. Assuming one parent is heterozygous for the disease and the other is normal, what is the probability of an affected individual having an affected child?

A One in two
B One in four
C One in eight
D One in 16
E One in 32

48 A number of cytogenetic methods can be employed in prenatal genetic screening. Which screening method examines interphase chromosomes?

A Agarose gel electrophoresis
B Fluorescence in situ hybridisation
C Multiplex ligation-dependent probe amplification
D Polymerase chain reaction
E Z-DNA isolation and amplification

49 During folliculogenesis, the oocyte is contained within a ball of cells. These cells are known as the:

A Basal lamina
B Granulosa
C Theca externa
D Theca interna
E Zona pellucida

50 At what stage of meiosis is the oocyte after ovulation?

A Anaphase I
B Metaphase I
C Metaphase II
D Prophase I
E Prophase II

51 Which cell type sits on the basement membrane of the seminiferous tubule and undergoes mitosis to generate cells that will ultimately develop into spermatozoa?

A Primary spermatocytes
B Secondary spermatocytes
C Sertoli cells
D Spermatids
E Spermatogonia

52 Following fertilisation, ion waves cause completion of the second meiotic division of the oocyte and fusion of cortical granules with the zona pellucida. Which ion is responsible?

A Ca^{2+}
B Cl^{-}
C HCO_3^{-}
D K^{+}
E Na^{+}

53 If a pregnant woman lies supine, she may experience a fall in blood pressure and feel dizzy and nauseous. What is the mechanism behind this phenomenon?

A Increased activation of the sympathetic nervous system
B Stimulation of the vagus nerve causing bradycardia
C The gravid uterus causes diaphragmatic splinting
D The gravid uterus compresses the aorta against the spine
E The gravid uterus compresses the inferior vena cava against the spine

54 What is the total extra iron requirement in pregnancy?

A 1 mg
B 10 mg
C 50 mg
D 100 mg
E 1000 mg

55 What are the most important hormones for the successful maintenance of lactation?

A Estrogen and oxytocin
B Estrogen and progesterone
C Estrogen and prolactin
D Prolactin and oxytocin
E Prolactin and progesterone

56 What is the name of the structure that shunts oxygenated blood from the right to left atrium in the fetus?

A Ductus arteriosus
B Ductus venosus
C Foramen ovale
D Ligamentum teres
E Pulmonary trunk

57 What compound forms the major constituent of pulmonary surfactant?

A Dipalmitoylphosphatidylcholine
B Surfactant-associated protein A
C Surfactant-associated protein D
D Phosphatidylcholine
E Phosphatidylglycerol

58 Fetal haemoglobin is more resistant to denaturation by acid and alkali than is adult haemoglobin. This principle forms the basis of which test that is used to estimate fetomaternal haemorrhage?

A Bohr test
B Coombs test
C Guthrie test
D Hamburger test
E Kleihauer test

59 From where in the kidney is renin secreted?

A Bowman's capsule
B Collecting ducts
C Distal convoluted tubule
D Juxtaglomerular cells
E Proximal convoluted tubule

60 Which cell type in the testis produces the majority of androgens?

A Leydig cells
B Myofibroblasts
C Sertoli cells
D Spermatocytes
E Spermatogonia

5 | Mock paper: paper 2

Answers to the questions in this chapter can be found in appendix 6.

1 What is the principle of DEXA scanning to assess bone mineral density?

A The absorption of a single high-dose X-ray beam is measured at two different angles
B The absorption of a single low-dose beam is measured at multiple intervals and analysed by a computer
C The absorption of a single low-dose X-ray beam is measured at two different angles
D Two high-dose X-ray beams are emitted and the absorption of the soft-tissue beam is subtracted from the total beam
E Two low-dose X-ray beams are emitted and the absorption of the soft-tissue beam is subtracted from the total beam

2 In radiotherapy, what is the SI unit of absorbed radiation dose?

A Curie
B Gray
C Joule
D Rad
E Sievert

3 What is the best description of the Doppler effect?

A A stationary target absorbs more ultrasound than a moving target
B A stationary target reflects more ultrasound than a moving target
C The frequency of a transmitted and reflected ultrasound wave are always constant
D The ultrasound wave reflected from a moving target has a different frequency from the transmitted wave
E The ultrasound wave reflected from a moving target has the same frequency as the transmitted wave

4 What are the advantages and disadvantages of resolution and penetration of transvaginal ultrasound (compared with transabdominal scanning)?

	Resolution	Penetration
A	Better	Greater
B	Better	Less
C	Worse	Greater
D	Worse	Less
E	Same	Same

5 A 67-year-old woman attends for a preoperative assessment. She has been taking furosemide for several years for hypertension. On questioning, she suffers from muscle cramps and constipation. What is the most likely electrolyte imbalance?

A Hypercalcaemia
B Hyperkalaemia
C Hypernatraemia
D Hypokalaemia
E Hyponatraemia

6 What percentage of hospital inpatients can expect to develop a hospital-acquired infection?

A 1%
B 2%
C 10%
D 20%
E 50%

7 Which gas is most commonly used for peritoneal insufflation in laparoscopy?

A Air
B Argon
C Carbon dioxide
D Nitrogen
E Oxygen

8 What is the principle underlying anti-D prophylaxis to prevent rhesus disease?

A Anti-D binds to rhesus-negative fetal erythrocytes in the maternal circulation, preventing sensitisation
B Anti-D binds to rhesus-negative maternal erythrocytes in the fetal circulation, preventing sensitisation
C Anti-D binds to rhesus-positive fetal erythrocytes in the maternal circulation, preventing sensitisation
D Anti-D binds to rhesus-positive maternal erythrocytes in the fetal circulation, preventing sensitisation
E Anti-D suppresses the maternal immune system

9 Which compound is useful in the prophylaxis and treatment of eclampsia?

A Magnesium chloride
B Magnesium hydroxide
C Magnesium sulphate
D Potassium chloride
E Potassium hydroxide

10 Following a forceps delivery, a woman is noted to have a perineal injury involving the external and internal anal sphincters as well as the anal epithelium. What degree of tear does she have?

A 2
B 3a
C 3b
D 3c
E 4

11 A 38-year-old woman has been referred to the gynaecology clinic with heavy menstrual bleeding. She has a BMI of 32 kg/m^2 and a previous history of a DVT. She has one child and is not sure if her family is complete. Her GP has prescribed tranexamic acid, but after reading the information leaflet she does not wish to take this drug. What is the most appropriate management?

A Cyclical norethisterone
B Insert a levonorgestrel-containing intrauterine system
C Mefenamic acid
D Transcervical resection of endometrium
E Vaginal hysterectomy

12 A junior doctor has carried out a research project in the early pregnancy unit. Low serum progesterone at six weeks of gestation has been evaluated for its ability to predict first-trimester miscarriage. Two hundred women were recruited. The results are as follows:

Serum progesterone	Miscarriage	Viable pregnancy
Low	60	40
Normal	20	80

What is the positive predictive value of low serum progesterone in predicting miscarriage?

A 20%
B 40%
C 50%
D 60%
E 80%

13 A woman sees her midwife for a routine antenatal check at 24 weeks of gestation. A urine dipstick is performed with the following results:

Protein	+
Ketones	–
Nitrites	+
Glucose	–

What is the appropriate course of action?

A Admit to hospital for IV antibiotics
B Arrange a 24-hour urine collection
C Commence oral antibiotics
D Reassure and do nothing
E Send urine for culture and microscopy

14 A white woman with type 2 diabetes attends the obstetric endocrine clinic at 16 weeks of gestation complaining of lethargy, weight gain and constipation. Thyroid function tests give the following results:

TSH	*10.2 mU/l (0.35–5.5 mU/l)*
Free T_4	*0.4 pmol/l (11–23 pmol/l)*
Thyroid peroxidase antibodies	*Positive*
Thyroid receptor antibodies	*Negative*

What is the most likely diagnosis?

A Graves' disease
B Hashimoto's thyroiditis
C Iodine deficiency
D Previous treatment with radioactive iodine
E Sheehan syndrome

15 What is the minimum volume of blood required to produce a pH and PCO_2 result in fetal blood sampling?

A 1 μl
B 5 μl
C 10 μl
D 25 μl
E 100 μl

16 Following a normal delivery, a baby has an Apgar score of 2 at 1 minute and 6 at 5 minutes. Cord blood samples are taken for gas analysis, with the following results:

	Umbilical artery	Umbilical vein
pH	7.28	7.35
PO_2 (kPa)	2.2	3.8
PCO_2 (kPa)	6.9	5.3
Base excess	−3	−2

What do the results show?

A Normal blood gases
B Significant fetal metabolic acidosis
C Significant fetal metabolic alkalosis
D Significant fetal respiratory acidosis
E Significant fetal respiratory alkalosis

17 What are the normal values of a cardiotocograph?

	Baseline heart rate	Baseline variability	Accelerations
A	110–160	0–4	>15 bpm for 15 seconds
B	110–160	>5	>15 bpm for 15 seconds
C	130–180	0–4	>30 bpm for 10 seconds
D	130–180	>5	>30 bpm for 10 seconds
E	>160	0–4	>15 bpm for 15 seconds

18 A 23-year-old presents to accident and emergency with sudden-onset left-sided abdominal pain. It is 17 days since her last menstrual period and she has a regular 28-day cycle. She is not using contraception. She is otherwise fit and well. An ultrasound scan is arranged with the following report:

> *Normal uterus and right ovary. In the left adnexa is a cystic structure measuring 3 × 4 cm with internal echoes in a reticular pattern and debris. There is a small amount of fluid in the pouch of Douglas.*

What is the most likely cause of her pain?

A Dermoid cyst
B Ectopic pregnancy
C Haemorrhagic cyst
D Ovarian carcinoma
E Ovarian torsion

19 In the new WHO manual for semen analysis, what is the minimum normal total sperm in the ejaculate?

A 15×10^6
B 20×10^6
C 32×10^6
D 39×10^6
E 50×10^6

20 A 25-year-old woman presents to her GP with an offensive off-white vaginal discharge. A sample of the discharge is sent to the microbiology laboratory, and the following report is returned:

> *Copious off-white discharge with pH 5.0. Amine test positive. On wet mount a large number of clue cells are seen.*

What is the most likely diagnosis?

A Bacterial vaginosis
B *Candida albicans* infection
C *Chlamydia trachomatis* infection
D Normal vaginal discharge
E *Trichomonas vaginalis* infection

21 A couple is referred to the fertility clinic with a two-year history of failure to conceive. The woman has irregular periods but is otherwise well. Basic tests are reported as follows:

FSH: 8.3 i.u./l (1–11 i.u./l)
Progesterone: 2.3 nmol/l (>30 nmol/l)
HSG: normal uterine cavity with bilateral tubal spill

Semen analysis:	*Count*	35×10^6/ml
	Progressive motility	*40%*
	Normal morphology	*10%*

What is the most likely cause of this couple's failure to conceive?

A Anovulation
B Asthenozoospermia
C Oligozoospermia
D Teratozoospermia
E Tubal disease

22 A woman is referred to the early pregnancy unit. It is 11 weeks since her last menstrual period and her pregnancy test is strongly positive. She has experienced some vaginal bleeding. An ultrasound scan is arranged with the following report:

> *Uterus larger than expected for dates. There is a gestational sac containing a fetus. The placenta is enlarged and thickened with numerous cystic spaces. Cysts identified on both ovaries. No free fluid.*

What is the most likely diagnosis?

A Complete molar pregnancy
B Ectopic pregnancy
C Heterotopic pregnancy
D Incomplete miscarriage
E Partial molar pregnancy

23 A woman who is eight weeks pregnant attends the early pregnancy unit with some vaginal bleeding. An ultrasound scan is arranged which shows a viable twin pregnancy with the following image:

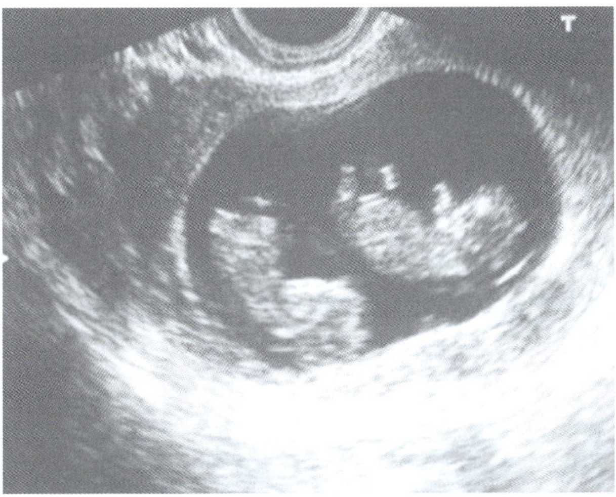

What is the chorionicity of these twins?

A Conjoined twins
B Dizygotic dichorionic diamniotic
C Monochorionic diamniotic
D Monozygotic dichorionic diamniotic
E Monochorionic monoamniotic

24 A 30-year-old woman attends the early pregnancy unit. It is six weeks since her last menstrual period and a pregnancy test is positive. She has had mild lower abdominal pain and has passed some brown vaginal discharge. The woman suffers with Crohn's disease and has a midline scar from a previous bowel resection. An ultrasound scan is arranged with the following report:

> *No intrauterine gestational sac identified. Both ovaries normal. No adnexal mass identified. No fluid seen in pouch of Douglas.*

A serum βhCG is 2800. A repeat serum βhCG 48 hours later is 3100.

What is the most appropriate management?

A Arrange a diagnostic laparoscopy
B Arrange an immediate laparotomy
C Discharge the patient
D Discuss treatment with methotrexate
E Repeat serum βhCG in 48 hours

25 Which class of immunoglobulin is primarily secreted in breast milk and protects the infant's intestinal mucosa from infection?

A IgA
B IgD
C IgE
D IgG
E IgM

26 Which type of immune hypersensitivity reaction best describes the condition of systemic lupus erythematosus?

A Type I (immediate) hypersensitivity
B Type II (antibody-mediated) hypersensitivity
C Type III (immune-complex) hypersensitivity
D Type IV (delayed-type) hypersensitivity
E Type V (suppressive-type) hypersensitivity

27 Which cell type is derived from monocytes and can trigger the adaptive immune response?

A Erythrocytes
B Macrophages
C Mast cells
D Mesangial cells
E Neutrophils

28 Which class I major histocompatibility complex human leucocyte antigen (HLA) is expressed only in extravillous trophoblast?

A HLA-A
B HLA-B
C HLA-C
D HLA-F
E HLA-G

29 Which pathogen is the causative agent in syphilis?

A *Candida albicans*
B *Chlamydia trachomatis*
C *Mycobacterium tuberculosis*
D *Neisseria gonorrhoeae*
E *Treponema pallidum*

30 Gestational maternal listeriosis can cause fetal infection with loss of the pregnancy. How does the pathogen responsible, *Listeria monocytogenes*, circumvent the immune system?

- A It can secrete dominant negative peptides which block MHC receptors
- B It can secrete porins which puncture and destroy plasma cells
- C It is an extracellular pathogen and uses host Fc receptors as decoys
- D It is an intracellular pathogen and 'hides' within phagocytic cells
- E It secretes defensins which prevent opsonisation

31 *Streptococcus* species of bacteria are the causative agents in many feto-maternal infections. What is the oxygen requirement for *Streptococcus*?

- A Definitive aerobe
- B Definitive anaerobe
- C Facultative anaerobe
- D Obligate aerobe
- E Obligate anaerobe

32 Which virus is responsible for chicken pox?

- A Cytomegalovirus
- B Herpes simplex virus
- C HIV
- D Parvovirus B19
- E Varicella-zoster virus

33 Through which route is cytomegalovirus infection most commonly transmitted?

- A Breastfeeding
- B Contact with saliva
- C Sexual contact
- D Sneezing
- E Social contact

34 To which family of viruses does the rubella virus belong?

A Adenoviruses
B Herpesviruses
C Poxviruses
D Retroviruses
E Togaviruses

35 Which animal is the primary host for the parasite *Toxoplasma gondii*?

A Bat
B Cat
C Cow
D Dog
E Pig

36 Which pathological term describes the reversible replacement of one differentiated cell type with another?

A Atrophy
B Dysplasia
C Hyperplasia
D Hypertrophy
E Metaplasia

37 In tuberculosis infection of the lung, the lung tissue can undergo necrosis with complete loss of tissue architecture. What pattern of necrosis is seen in pulmonary tuberculosis infection?

A Caseous necrosis
B Coagulative necrosis
C Fibrinoid necrosis
D Gangrenous necrosis
E Liquefactive necrosis

38 Which two inflammatory mediators are released by both mast cells and platelets?

A Cytokines and leucotrienes
B Cytokines and nitric oxide
C Histamine and leucotrienes
D Histamine and prostaglandins
E Histamine and serotonin

39 During embryogenesis, there may be programmed cell death, which is necessary for the correct development of anatomical structures. What is the correct pathological term for this?

A Apoptosis
B Atrophy
C Karyolysis
D Karyorrhexis
E Necrosis

40 During the process of wound healing, which cell type migrates into the wound area and secretes extracellular matrix and collagen?

A Fibroblasts
B Lymphocytes
C Macrophages
D Monocytes
E Neutrophils

41 What type of compound is bradykinin?

A Glycoprotein
B Leucotriene
C Peptide
D Prostaglandin
E Steroid

42 What is the pathological term for a malignancy of mesenchymal origin?

A Carcinoma
B Choristoma
C Hamartoma
D Sarcoma
E Teratoma

43 Choriocarcinoma is a malignant form of gestational trophoblastic disease. When choriocarcinoma metastasises, it has a propensity for which type of spread?

A Haematogenous
B Implantation
C Lymphatic
D Transcoelomic
E Transplantation

44 Hereditary non-polyposis colorectal cancer (Lynch syndrome) demonstrates which type of inheritance?

A Autosomal dominant
B Autosomal recessive
C X-linked dominant
D X-linked recessive
E Y-linked dominant

45 Which paraneoplastic syndromes are associated with small cell carcinoma of the lung?

A Acanthosis nigricans and carcinoid syndrome
B Polycythaemia and acanthosis nigricans
C Polycythaemia and Cushing syndrome
D SIADH and carcinoid syndrome
E SIADH and Cushing syndrome

46 What type of fibroid is indicated by X in the diagram below?

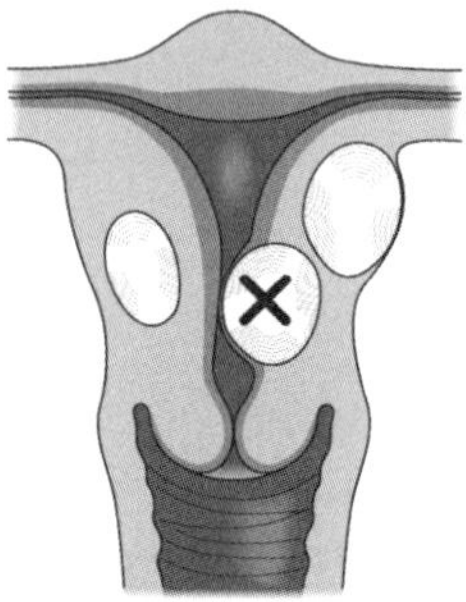

A Cervical
B Intramural
C Pedunculated
D Submucous
E Subserous

47 Tamoxifen is a selective estrogen receptor modulator that is used in the treatment of breast cancer. Prolonged tamoxifen use is associated with an increased risk of which gynaecological cancer?

A Cervical
B Endometrial
C Fallopian tube
D Ovarian
E Vulval

48 The Pearl index is commonly used to report the effectiveness of a contraceptive method. How is it calculated?

A Months of exposure / number of pregnancies
B Months of exposure / number of pregnancies × 100
C Months of exposure / number of pregnancies × 1200
D Number of pregnancies / months of exposure × 100
E Number of pregnancies / months of exposure × 1200

49 Which compound constitutes the estrogenic component of the majority of combined oral contraceptive pills?

A Estradiol
B Estriol
C Estrone
D Ethinylestradiol
E Tibolone

50 Ulipristal acetate is a drug used for emergency contraception. What class of drug is ulipristal acetate?

A Aromatase inhibitor
B Estrogen antagonist
C Progesterone antagonist
D Selective estrogen receptor modulator
E Selective progesterone receptor modulator

51 What is the mechanism of action of hydralazine?

A $\alpha 2$ agonist
B Angiotensin-converting enzyme inhibitor
C Antimuscarinic
D $\beta 2$ agonist
E Direct-acting smooth-muscle relaxant

52 In utero exposure to warfarin can result in warfarin embryopathy (fetal warfarin syndrome). Exposure at which weeks of gestation is most likely to lead to this condition?

A 6–9/40
B 12–14/40
C 18–20/40
D 24–26/40
E 32–36/40

53 Clavulanic acid and sulbactam are examples of which class of drugs?

A Aminoglycosides
B Betalactamase inhibitors
C Cephalosporins
D Macrolides
E Penicillins

54 Fentanyl is a strong agonist at which type of opioid receptor?

A α (alpha)
B δ (delta)
C κ (kappa)
D μ (mu)
E Nociceptin receptor

55 Ondansetron is an effective antiemetic. It is an antagonist at which receptor?

A 5-HT1a
B 5-HT3
C D2
D H1
E H2

56 What type of membrane ion channel is blocked by verapamil?

A Bicarbonate
B Calcium
C Chloride
D Potassium
E Sodium

57 Which enzyme is blocked by acetazolamide?

A Angiotensin-converting enzyme
B Carbonic anhydrase
C Cyclooxygenase
D Glutaminase
E Penicillinase

58 Which class of drugs is antagonised by flumazenil?

A Antiemetics
B Antipsychotics
C Benzodiazepines
D Neuroleptics
E Opiates

59 Anticonvulsant drugs are known to have harmful effects on the developing fetus. Which single agent is associated with the greatest risk?

A Carbamazepine
B Gabapentin
C Lamotrigine
D Levetiracetam
E Sodium valproate

60 A woman attends for her antenatal booking visit and it is noted that she is taking unbranded multivitamins purchased from a supermarket. Which vitamin may be embryotoxic if the dosage is too high?

A Vitamin A
B Vitamin B_{12}
C Vitamin C
D Vitamin E
E Vitamin K

Appendix 1
Blueprinting matrix for the Part 1 MRCOG examination

GLOBAL		UNDERSTANDING CELL FUNCTION			UNDERSTANDING HUMAN STRUCTURE			
	MODULE	Physiology	Endocrinology	Biochemistry	Anatomy	Embryology	Genetics	Biophysic
1	Clinical skills	Understand the physiological basis of physical signs in obstetrics and gynaecology.					Structure and function of chromosomes and genes. Genomics and regulation of gene expression.	
3	IT, clinical governance and research							
5	Core surgical skills	Physiology of wound healing. Physiology of major organ systems as applied to surgical practice. Fluid and electrolyte balance in the perioperative period. Nutritional physiology in health and disease. Principles of blood transfusion.	Mechanisms of hormone action. Hormone types. Perioperative care and common endocrino-pathies (e.g. diabetes and thyroid disorders). Effects of anaesthesia and surgery on endocrine homeostasis and fluid balance.	Structure and function of normal cells. Biochemistry of catabolism and nutrition as applied to surgery. Biochemistry of enzymes, vitamins and minerals. Effects of surgery on the fetus.	Surgical anatomy of the pelvis and abdomen. Detailed functional anatomy of abdominal wall, abdominal cavity and pelvis, their contents, relevant bones, joints, muscles, blood vessels, lymphatics, nerve supply and histology. Understanding of breast and end	Developmental abnormalities in the female. Development of the urogenital tract and structural abnormalities. Structural abnormalities in the female reproductuve tract.	Structure and function of chromosomes and genes.	Principles o electro-cardiograph ultrasound, Doppler, X-rays and MR Use of laser and electrosurge

ERSTANDING MEASUREMENT AND MANIPULATION			UNDERSTANDING ILLNESS			
pidemiology and statistics	**Data interpretation**	**Pharmacology**	**Immunology**	**Microbiology**	**Pathology**	**Clinical management**
nciples of e indications, ks, benefits d fectiveness of vestigations.	Principles of fluid and electrolyte and acid–base balance. Interpret results of investigations including microbiology swabs, haematological tests and electrolyte levels.	Safe prescribing, avoiding drug errors, drug interactions, adverse effects.			Understand the pathological basis of physical signs.	Analyse an obstetric and gynaecological history. Understand the principles underpinning clinical examinations. Aware of Fraser competence issue.
rinciples of creening. tatistical ethods used in inical research. rinciples of inical trial esign. nderstand udit cycle and ifference from esearch. Levels f evidence, uantification of sk and chance.	Understand accuracy of tests used in diagnosis.	Comparison of effectiveness/ cost-effectiveness, number needed to treat.				
pidemiology f surgical omplications. rinciples of nformed onsent.	Methods of measurement and interpretation of clinically important physiological variables as applied to surgical practice.	Pharmacokinetics and factors affecting drug action.	Organisation of immune system, immunogenetics and principles of antigen recognition. Immunology of graft rejection and immune responses in infection, inflammation and trauma.	Biology of microorganisms encountered in surgical practice. Principles of infection control. Principles of antimicrobial prophylaxis and wound care.	Understand the histopathology of the pelvic organs, the breast and the endocrine organs, including the pituitary and the hypothalamus.	You will be expected to demonstrate knowledge of the principles underpinning fluid and electrolyte balance, and coagulation. You will be expected to demonstrate knowledge of the basic clinical skills in core surgical practice.

GLOBAL		UNDERSTANDING CELL FUNCTION			UNDERSTANDING HUMAN STRUCTURE			
	MODULE	Physiology	Endocrinology	Biochemistry	Anatomy	Embryology	Genetics	Biophysic
6	Post-operative care							
7	Surgical procedures						Diagnosis of fetal abnormalities.	
8	Antenatal care	Physiology of pregnancy including acid–base, fluid and electrolyte balance in healthy and pathological pregnancy. Fetal physiology and its development with fetal growth. Cellular physiology of the major organ systems in the non-pregnant woman.	Endocrinology of pregnancy. The placenta as an endocrine gland.	Placental transfer.	Anatomical adaptations to pregnancy. Breast changes in pregnancy. Anatomical interpretation of fetal and maternal images from X-ray, ultrasound and magnetic resonance imaging.	Fetal embryology.	Chromosomal and genetic disorders – principles of inheritance. Features and effects of common inherited disorders and origins of fetal malformation.	
9	Maternal medicine	Physiology in disorders of pregnancy.	Diabetes in pregnancy. Pituitary, thyroid, adrenal and other endocrine disorders relevant to pregnancy.	Cellular biochemistry in disorders of pregnancy.		Fetal and placental growth and development – particularly neural tube, gut and cardiac development.	Genetic principles underlying screening for fetal anomaly.	Physics of Doppler, ultrasound and magentic resonance imaging.

DERSTANDING MEASUREMENT AND MANIPULATION			UNDERSTANDING ILLNESS			
Epidemiology and statistics	Data interpretation	Pharmacology	Immunology	Microbiology	Pathology	Clinical management
ctors affecting rgical rates, erative ccess and mplication tes.		Properties and actions of drugs used after surgery. Antibiotics and antibiotic prophylaxis.				You should be able to show understanding of the management surrounding surgical complications, infection and infection control.
		Properties and actions of drugs, including anaesthetic agents used during surgery. Effect of drugs on haemostasis and uterine bleeding.				Principles of procedures used in surgical practice.
rinciples of creening. creening in regnancy for etal disorders. pidemiology of isorders and omplications of pregnancy. ou should be ble to define nd interpret data on eonatal and erinatal nortality.	Interpret commonly performed tests in pregnancy including screening tests. Interpret data on maternal mortality.	Prescribing in pregnancy. Placental handling of drugs. Effects of drugs on the pregnant woman and fetus. Drugs for fetal development and wellbeing.	Maternofetal immunology.	Infection in pregnancy. Screening for infection. Virus biology.	Effect of pregnancy on disease and disease on pregnancy. Teratogenesis.	Principles underlying the management of common disorders of pregnancy.
Definitions of maternal, neonatal and perinatal mortality and their interpretation.	Interpret commonly performed tests in maternal medicine.	Drugs and their adverse effects in pregnancy. Drugs used in pregnancy-specific pathologies and complications of pregnancy.	Immunology of pregnancy. The fetus as an allograft. Isoimmunisation.	Infectious complications of pregnancy and their management. Fetal impact of maternal infection.		Principles underlying the management of common disorders of pregnancy complicated by maternal disease.

GLOBAL		UNDERSTANDING CELL FUNCTION			UNDERSTANDING HUMAN STRUCTURE			
	MODULE	Physiology	Endocrinology	Biochemistry	Anatomy	Embryology	Genetics	Biophysics
10	Management of labour	Physiology of parturition, myometrial contractility and cervical dilatation. Fetal physiology in late pregnancy and during labour, including methods of assessment of fetal wellbeing.	Endocrinology of parturition. Development and maturation of the fetal endocrine system.	Biochemistry of prosta-glandins and steroid hormones. Hormones, receptors and intracellular signalling. Biochemistry of myometrial contractility.	Obstetric anatomy of the pelvis and abdomen. Changes during late pregnancy and in labour. Mechanism of childbirth.			
11	Management of delivery	Physiology of the third stage of labour.		Acid–base balance.				
12	Postpartum problems	Lactation and uterine involution.	Endocrinology of lactation.		Structural changes in the newborn.			
13	Gynae-cological problems	Physiology of the reproductive tract in women.	Menopause and endocrine effects on bone, vasomotor system, etc. Puberty and growth. Menstrual cycle.		Gynaecological anatomy.	Development of the reproductive tract.	Chromosome abnormalities, single gene disorders, sex-linked inheritance.	

ERSTANDING MEASUREMENT AND MANIPULATION			UNDERSTANDING ILLNESS			
Epidemiology and statistics	Data interpretation	Pharmacology	Immunology	Microbiology	Pathology	Clinical management
	Interpret commonly performed tests in labour including fetal blood sampling.	Tocolysis and stimulants of uterine contractility. Pain relief in labour and the puerperium.		Infection and its management in labour and delivery.		Understand the principles of management of labour.
	Interpret cord blood samples.	Drugs in management of delivery. Third stage of labour and its problems. Effects of drugs on the newborn.			Placental site and implantation and its abnormalities.	Understand the principles of operative delivery and perineal tear.
		Contraception in the postpartum period. Use of drugs during lactation.		Puerperal sepsis. Infection and its management in the postpartum period.		Understand the principles of management of postpartum problems, including haemorrhage.
pidemiology f common ynaecological nditions.	Interpret commonly performed investigations for benign gynaecological conditions.	Drugs in benign gynaecology, including treatment of menorrhagia, dysmenorrhoea, endometriosis, polycystic ovary syndrome, menopause, osteoporosis.	Immunology of tissue grafting and graft rejection. Immune responses to infection, inflammation and trauma. Graft-versus-host reaction, autoimmunity, immunisation and immuno-suppression.	Infectious diseases in gynaecological practice.	Congenital abnormalities of the genital tract. Osteopenia/ osteoporosis. Pathological conditions of the uterus (endometrium and myometrium), tubes and ovaries.	Understand the principles of management of common gynaecological problems.

GLOBAL		UNDERSTANDING CELL FUNCTION			UNDERSTANDING HUMAN STRUCTURE			
	MODULE	Physiology	Endocrinology	Biochemistry	Anatomy	Embryology	Genetics	Biophysic
14	Subfertility	Physiology of the reproductive tract in men and women. Regulation of spermato-genesis, fertilisation and establishment of early pregnancy.	Endocrinology of the H-P-O axis. Endocrino-pathies leading to anovulation in PCOS, hypogonadal hypogonadism, hyper-prolactinaemia and premature ovarian failure.		Anatomy of the hypothalamus and pituitary, and the male and female reproductive organs. Surgical anatomy of the pelvis and abdomen.	Development of the gametes, fertilisation, implantation and early embryonic development. Regulation of the embryonic genome. Development of the reproductive tract.	Congenital abnormalities leading to infertility.	Use of transvagina and transabdom ultrasound. X-ray and hysterosalp gography.
15	Sexual and reproductive health	The impact of contraceptives on the physiology of the reproductive tract.	Interactions between hormonal contraceptives and endocrine physiology.					
16	Early pregnancy care	Luteoplacental shift and fetomaternal communi-cation.	Maternal recognition of pregnancy, endocrinology of the corpus luteum and early pregnancy.	Hormonal changes associated with pregnancy loss.		Chromosomal abnormalities associated with pregnancy loss.		Ultrasound in early pregnancy.
17	Gynae-cological oncology	Physiology in gynaecological oncology.	Hormome-secreting and hormone-dependent tumours in gynaecology.	Regulation of the cell cycle. Cell biology in gynae-cological cancer.	Anatomical changes relevant to tumours in the female.		Genetic origins of cancer and DNA mutations. Principles of molecular testing for gynaecological cancers.	Physics of laser and MRI. Principles o radiotherap
18	Urogynae-cology and pelvic floor problems	Physiology of the kidney and urinary tract.			Functional anatomy of the pelvic floor, kidney and urinary tract.	Congenital abnormalities of the renal tract.		Principles o measuremer of bladder function.

...ERSTANDING MEASUREMENT AND MANIPULATION			UNDERSTANDING ILLNESS			
...pidemiology and statistics	Data interpretation	Pharmacology	Immunology	Microbiology	Pathology	Clinical management
...idemiology of ...ertility.	Interpret basic investigations for infertility.	Drugs used to treat infertility. Drugs used in anovulation, superovulation and assisted conception. Drug teratogenicity.	Principles of reproductive immunology.	Pelvic inflammatory disease and its effects on fertility.	Pathology of tubal damage, polycystic ovary syndrome, endometriosis and the pituitary. Histology and pathology of the male genital tract.	Understand the principles of management of subfertility.
...idemiology of ...ntraception ...d STIs.	Interpret results of investigations for genital tract infection.	Contraceptives. Drugs used for medical termination of pregnancy. Drugs used for STIs, including antimicrobial resistance.		Sexually transmitted infections.	Pathological features of STD and female genital infections. Endometrial effects of contraceptive steroids.	Understand the principles of management of STD. Understand the prescribing of contraception.
...idemiology of ...egnancy ...ilure.	Interpret ultrasound in early pregnancy and commonly performed investigations including hCG measurement.	Medical management of miscarriage, trophoblastic disease and ectopic pregnancy.	Immunology of pregnancy and miscarriage.	Infective factors predisposing to pregnancy loss and ectopic pregnancy.	Pathology of miscarriage, ectopic pregnancy, trophoblastic disease.	Understand the principles of management of early pregnancy failure.
...idemiology of ...ncers affecting ...omen.		Properties and actions of drugs used to treat gynaecological cancers and trophoblastic disorders. Effects of chemotherapeutic agents on gonadal function.	Tumour surveillance and immunotherapy.	HPV and other viral origins of cancer.	Pathology, histology and classification of gynaecological cancers and premalignant conditions. Field change effects. Aetiological factors. Cervical cytology. Pathology of pain and transmission of pain signals centrally.	Understand the principles of management of gynaecological cancer.
		Properties and actions of drugs used in urogynaecology.		Urinary tract infection.	Pathological conditions of the bladder, urethra and vagina.	Understand the principles of management of disorders of the urinary tract and perineum.

Appendix 2
Example SBA answer sheet

The Royal College of Obstetricians and Gynaecologists

Part 1 Membership Examination – Paper 1 – SBA Answer Sheet

Surname (Family Name)

Other Name(s)

This form will be read by a machine
Please use an HB pencil provided.
Mark each answer with a single horizontal line A B C
If you make a mistake erase it completely
Do NOT mark with ticks, crosses or circles
Do NOT forget to enter your name and candidate number properly

Candidate Number

0	0	0	0
1	1	1	1
2	2	2	2
3	3	3	3
4	4	4	4
5	5	5	5
6	6	6	6
7	7	7	7
8	8	8	8
9	9	9	9

1 A B C D E	21 A B C D E	41 A B C D E
2 A B C D E	22 A B C D E	42 A B C D E
3 A B C D E	23 A B C D E	43 A B C D E
4 A B C D E	24 A B C D E	44 A B C D E
5 A B C D E	25 A B C D E	45 A B C D E
6 A B C D E	26 A B C D E	46 A B C D E
7 A B C D E	27 A B C D E	47 A B C D E
8 A B C D E	28 A B C D E	48 A B C D E
9 A B C D E	29 A B C D E	49 A B C D E
10 A B C D E	30 A B C D E	50 A B C D E
11 A B C D E	31 A B C D E	51 A B C D E
12 A B C D E	32 A B C D E	52 A B C D E
13 A B C D E	33 A B C D E	53 A B C D E
14 A B C D E	34 A B C D E	54 A B C D E
15 A B C D E	35 A B C D E	55 A B C D E
16 A B C D E	36 A B C D E	56 A B C D E
17 A B C D E	37 A B C D E	57 A B C D E
18 A B C D E	38 A B C D E	58 A B C D E
19 A B C D E	39 A B C D E	59 A B C D E
20 A B C D E	40 A B C D E	60 A B C D E

The Royal College of Obstetricians and Gynaecologists

Part 1 Membership Examination – Paper 1 – MCQ Answer Sheet

This form will be read by a machine
Please use an HB pencil provided.
Mark each answer with a single horizontal line T for True and F for False
If you make a mistake erase it completely
Do NOT mark with ticks, crosses or circles
Do NOT forget to enter your name and candidate number properly

	A	B	C	D	E		A	B	C	D	E
61	T F	T F	T F	T F	T F	76	T F	T F	T F	T F	T F
62	T F	T F	T F	T F	T F	77	T F	T F	T F	T F	T F
63	T F	T F	T F	T F	T F	78	T F	T F	T F	T F	T F
64	T F	T F	T F	T F	T F	79	T F	T F	T F	T F	T F
65	T F	T F	T F	T F	T F	80	T F	T F	T F	T F	T F
66	T F	T F	T F	T F	T F	81	T F	T F	T F	T F	T F
67	T F	T F	T F	T F	T F	82	T F	T F	T F	T F	T F
68	T F	T F	T F	T F	T F	83	T F	T F	T F	T F	T F
69	T F	T F	T F	T F	T F	84	T F	T F	T F	T F	T F
70	T F	T F	T F	T F	T F	85	T F	T F	T F	T F	T F
71	T F	T F	T F	T F	T F	86	T F	T F	T F	T F	T F
72	T F	T F	T F	T F	T F	87	T F	T F	T F	T F	T F
73	T F	T F	T F	T F	T F	88	T F	T F	T F	T F	T F
74	T F	T F	T F	T F	T F	89	T F	T F	T F	T F	T F
75	T F	T F	T F	T F	T F	90	T F	T F	T F	T F	T F

Appendix 3
Answers to chapter 2 questions

SBA 1	A
SBA 2	E
SBA 3	A
SBA 4	A
SBA 5	B
SBA 6	C
SBA 7	B
SBA 8	E
SBA 9	E
SBA 10	C
SBA 11	B
SBA 12	B
SBA 13	D
SBA 14	C
SBA 15	E
SBA 16	A
SBA 17	B
SBA 18	D
SBA 19	C
SBA 20	C
SBA 21	D
SBA 22	E
SBA 23	D
SBA 24	E
SBA 25	C
SBA 26	C
SBA 27	E
SBA 28	B
SBA 29	B
SBA 30	E
SBA 31	E
SBA 32	A
SBA 33	A
SBA 34	D
SBA 35	D
SBA 36	A
SBA 37	E
SBA 38	C
SBA 39	B
SBA 40	C
SBA 41	B
SBA 42	D
SBA 43	D
SBA 44	E
SBA 45	A
SBA 46	B
SBA 47	A
SBA 48	C
SBA 49	B
SBA 50	B
SBA 51	C
SBA 52	A
SBA 53	A
SBA 54	C
SBA 55	E
SBA 56	E
SBA 57	A
SBA 58	B
SBA 59	A
SBA 60	C
SBA 61	D
SBA 62	C
SBA 63	E
SBA 64	A

Appendix 4
Answers to chapter 3 questions

SBA 65 ▶ E
SBA 66 ▶ D
SBA 67 ▶ E
SBA 68 ▶ A
SBA 69 ▶ B
SBA 70 ▶ A
SBA 71 ▶ A
SBA 72 ▶ D
SBA 73 ▶ C
SBA 74 ▶ E
SBA 75 ▶ A
SBA 76 ▶ D
SBA 77 ▶ B
SBA 78 ▶ E
SBA 79 ▶ B
SBA 80 ▶ A
SBA 81 ▶ B
SBA 82 ▶ B
SBA 83 ▶ B
SBA 84 ▶ B
SBA 85 ▶ E
SBA 86 ▶ D
SBA 87 ▶ A
SBA 88 ▶ B
SBA 89 ▶ C
SBA 90 ▶ C
SBA 91 ▶ C
SBA 92 ▶ E
SBA 93 ▶ E
SBA 94 ▶ A
SBA 95 ▶ C
SBA 96 ▶ A
SBA 97 ▶ C
SBA 98 ▶ E
SBA 99 ▶ E
SBA 100 ▶ E
SBA 101 ▶ B
SBA 102 ▶ D
SBA 103 ▶ C
SBA 104 ▶ E
SBA 105 ▶ E
SBA 106 ▶ D
SBA 107 ▶ A
SBA 108 ▶ C
SBA 109 ▶ E
SBA 110 ▶ C
SBA 111 ▶ C
SBA 112 ▶ B
SBA 113 ▶ A
SBA 114 ▶ D
SBA 115 ▶ B
SBA 116 ▶ D
SBA 117 ▶ A
SBA 118 ▶ D
SBA 119 ▶ D
SBA 120 ▶ C
SBA 121 ▶ D
SBA 122 ▶ D
SBA 123 ▶ E
SBA 124 ▶ B
SBA 125 ▶ A
SBA 126 ▶ B
SBA 127 ▶ C
SBA 128 ▶ C
SBA 129 ▶ E
SBA 130 ▶ D
SBA 131 ▶ A
SBA 132 ▶ C
SBA 133 ▶ B
SBA 134 ▶ B
SBA 135 ▶ A
SBA 136 ▶ A
SBA 137 ▶ D
SBA 138 ▶ A
SBA 139 ▶ E
SBA 140 ▶ A

Appendix 5
Answers to mock paper 1 (chapter 4)

1	▶	C
2	▶	E
3	▶	C
4	▶	D
5	▶	A
6	▶	C
7	▶	A
8	▶	A
9	▶	B
10	▶	C
11	▶	D
12	▶	C
13	▶	A
14	▶	D
15	▶	E
16	▶	C
17	▶	D
18	▶	C
19	▶	D
20	▶	E
21	▶	C
22	▶	C
23	▶	A
24	▶	E
25	▶	D
26	▶	C
27	▶	C
28	▶	B
29	▶	A
30	▶	E
31	▶	A
32	▶	B
33	▶	A
34	▶	A
35	▶	D
36	▶	B
37	▶	C
38	▶	D
39	▶	C
40	▶	A
41	▶	D
42	▶	E
43	▶	B
44	▶	D
45	▶	E
46	▶	B
47	▶	A
48	▶	B
49	▶	B
50	▶	C
51	▶	E
52	▶	A
53	▶	E
54	▶	E
55	▶	D
56	▶	C
57	▶	A
58	▶	E
59	▶	D
60	▶	A

Appendix 6
Answers to mock paper 2 (chapter 5)

1 ▶ E
2 ▶ B
3 ▶ D
4 ▶ B
5 ▶ D
6 ▶ C
7 ▶ C
8 ▶ C
9 ▶ C
10 ▶ E
11 ▶ B
12 ▶ D
13 ▶ E
14 ▶ B
15 ▶ D
16 ▶ A
17 ▶ B
18 ▶ C
19 ▶ D
20 ▶ A
21 ▶ A
22 ▶ E
23 ▶ C
24 ▶ D
25 ▶ A
26 ▶ C
27 ▶ B
28 ▶ E
29 ▶ E
30 ▶ D
31 ▶ C
32 ▶ E
33 ▶ A
34 ▶ E
35 ▶ B
36 ▶ E
37 ▶ A
38 ▶ E
39 ▶ A
40 ▶ A
41 ▶ C
42 ▶ D
43 ▶ A
44 ▶ A
45 ▶ E
46 ▶ D
47 ▶ B
48 ▶ E
49 ▶ D
50 ▶ E
51 ▶ E
52 ▶ A
53 ▶ B
54 ▶ D
55 ▶ B
56 ▶ B
57 ▶ B
58 ▶ C
59 ▶ E
60 ▶ A